YOGA BODY, BUDDHA MIND

YOGA BODY, BUDDHA MIND

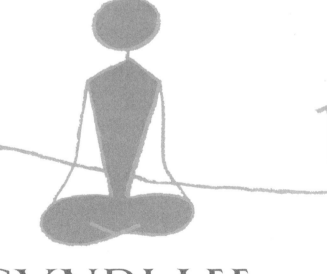

CYNDI LEE

RIVERHEAD BOOKS, NEW YORK

RIVERHEAD BOOKS
Published by The Berkley Publishing Group
A division of Penguin Group (USA) Inc.
375 Hudson Street
New York, New York 10014

Copyright © 2004 by Cyndi Lee
Interior photographs by David Bartolomi
Cover and interior illustrations by Cyndi Lee

First Riverhead trade paperback edition: August 2004

Library of Congress Cataloging-in-Publication Data

Lee, Cyndi.
    Yoga body, Buddha mind / Cyndi Lee.
        p. cm.
    ISBN 1-59448-024-9
    1. Yoga, Haòha—Handbooks, manuals, etc.   2. Exercise—Handbooks, manuals, etc.
3. Health—Handbooks, manuals, etc.   I. Title.

RA781.7.L438 2004
613.7'046—dc22

                                                                2004046793

Printed in the United States of America

10   9   8   7   6   5   4

For all my teachers,
especially Gehlek Rimpoche and Chogyam Trungpa Rinpoche

and

for all my students,
especially the OMmies

ACKNOWLEDGMENTS

Thank you to Melvin McLeod—without his initial encouragement, generosity, and guidance as well as the opportunity to write a yoga column in the *Shambhala Sun* for the past three years, this book would not exist.

Way back when, my dear student Jean Gallagher, who is a writing teacher and poet, read my first little work in progress. She helped me make it so much better, and she liked it! To her I make a low gassho.

I am very grateful to Shayna Samuels for actually putting me on a schedule, nudging me about deadlines, and then editing the whole book twice before it even went to the publisher.

Much appreciation to my patient and supportive editor, Amy Hertz, for her passion for yoga, dharma sisterhood, and two crucial pieces of advice that were just what I needed. Her assistant, Marc Haeringer, has been so helpful every step of the way.

A huge thank-you to my agent, Sarah Jane Freyman, who told me there was a book inside me and gave me the tools to unearth it.

Hugs and bows to Catherine Lippincott, publicist and yogini, and Brian Liem, OM Yoga Center's director of programming as well as an OM yoga teacher, for being the yoga models in this book. Margi Young and Jennifer Brilliant were the sharp and kind eagle eyes for our asanas.

I offer sincere thanks to the fine, committed, and talented yoga teachers at

OM Yoga Center who use their hearts and hands in equal measure to share this practice of yoga and Buddhist teachings with all of our students.

Thank you also to all the front desk folks and those who have held down the fort in the back office each time I vanished to work on this book.

The people at OM that play the part of students are truly why OM is a home and a family. We have been through so much together and I can never express how much you all mean to me. Thanks for letting me try out all these stories on you and for coming along on the ride.

I have been extremely fortunate to learn about yoga and life from many teachers and I am grateful to them all, especially the sweet and smart Judith Lasater and the masterful Rodney Yee.

I thank my dear dad for a talent for movement, a knack for communicating, and a spiritual yearning that shows up as joy. He inspired me always. I thank my mom for her quiet and steady support—it gives me confidence and comfort.

David Nichtern is not just my number one advisor and most excellent husband, but a brilliant dharma teacher who introduced me to the teachings of Chogyam Trungpa and changed my life forever. Thank you for meeting my mind again and again and again.

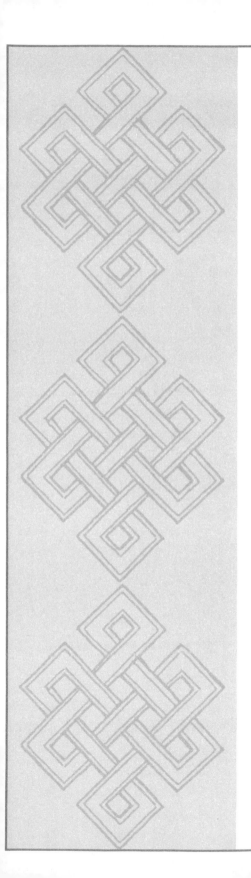

CONTENTS

ONE
AWAKENED UNION
Body, Breath, and Mind

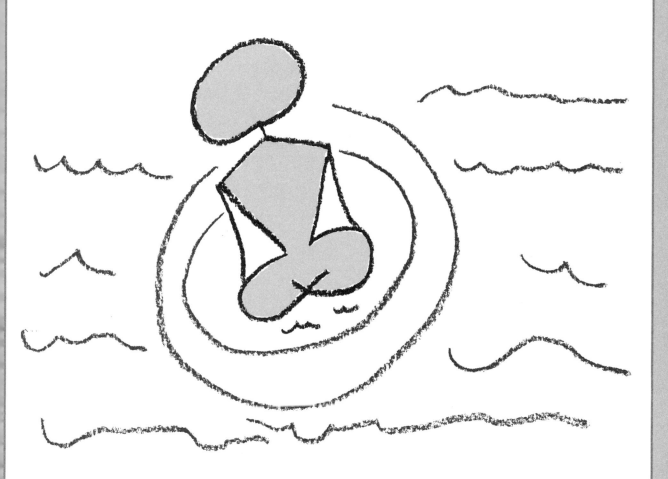

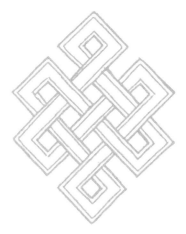

It came without warning right at the beginning of the day trip down the river. I really don't like water, and I am a weak, underconfident swimmer at best. But people I trusted said it was fun and not scary at all. If you did fall out, you would land on a little rock and immediately be picked up in the next boat. So I went and on the very first bend in the river, I slid out. There was no warning and no big inhale before plunging into icy cold, wildly churning water. And then there I was, trapped under a rubber boat in the whitewater rapids of the Pacuare River in Costa Rica.

No breath in my lungs and nobody can see where I am. I thought, "Wow, this is how it happens," and I visualized a small article in the *New York Times*—"Yoga Teacher Drowns While Leading Retreat in Costa Rica." My mind raced and my lungs got tight but, somehow, I didn't panic.

The yoga, breathing, and meditation practices that I had been doing for years prepared me for that very moment. Breath awareness, manipulation, and retention practice allowed me to intuitively know that I could go without breath for way longer than was comfortable. My daily twisting and inverting enabled me to know what was up and down and to maintain a highly fluid sense of balance. Meditation had trained me to stay focused on the task at hand, even while thoughts of my own death were running rampant through my head. I groped my way along the bottom of the boat and popped up into the rapids.

A very long minute later, a bodybuilder/yoga student floated by, grabbed me by the collar, and plopped me into his boat. Gehlek Rimpoche, a Tibetan lama, had taught me that to meet the teachings of the Buddha in your lifetime is as fortunate and rare as a tortoise's head popping up into an inner tube in the middle of the ocean. In that moment I felt just like that tortoise. Sitting in the haven of boat #2, my heart hammering, my adrenaline rushing, my lungs gasping, I was as scared as I've ever been. But when I was under the boat I was not scared. I was wide awake, balanced, and steady. Mindfulness meditation, yoga postures, and breath awareness are all powerful practices that can affect our lives deeply, but there is no doubt in my mind that in this life-threatening moment, it was the combination of all three that saved my life.

I am passionate about yoga and have been fortunate to share it with many students over the past twenty years. I have been a student of Tibetan Buddhism for more than ten years and it has been a natural evolution for the two lineages to merge in my teaching. Yoga and Buddhism offer insights and experiences that complement each other and together complete a basic homework assignment for humans—what do I do with this body and this mind?

MEDITATION

Back in 1972 I started taking yoga classes for an easy P.E. credit in college. The feeling of being cleansed, like taking a shower from the inside out, was unmatched by any other kind of exercise I had experienced and that is still true for me today, even after twenty years of professional dancing. My teachers were inspiring and I was highly motivated. It didn't take long for me to be able to hold my breath for over a minute, or to stand on my head for five minutes. I was hooked.

But I got left behind when it came to the "spiritual" part. I just didn't get it, or, as a friend of mine said, it didn't get me. My teachers quoted Patanjali, author of the Yoga Sutra, who wrote, "Yoga is the cessation of the fluctuations of the mind." Then they turned off the lights and said, "Close your eyes and don't move a muscle." They sat up very erect, shut their lids, and seemed to somehow plug into a big bliss cloud of happiness. I tried it, too, but my mind did not cease to fluctuate. I had many thoughts and not all of them were happy. After all the detailed instructions about how to work with my body, I felt abandoned by the lack of information relating to my mind. I did my best to try to feel at least pleasant, but then the class was over. Walking down the street, my body was strong, clean, juicy, and open, but I felt inadequate and cranky.

It turns out that my experience wasn't that unusual. While most people do walk out of yoga class in better physical shape than when they walked in, their personal awakening may still be elusive. Practicing yoga postures is an unparalleled method of strengthening muscles, enhancing breathing, cleansing toxins, and soothing the nervous system, but the sense of harmonious rejuvenation that arises by the end of the class may quickly dissipate once our feet hit the pavement in front of the yoga studio door. People's bodies will change but their mind will still be jumping, their heart still buried under layers of tension and fear.

As a teacher, I have seen again and again that if you are a type A personality, you will do your yoga practice with the same aggression and competitiveness that shapes the rest of your life. If you are sloppy, your posture will reflect that. If you are easily frustrated, that tendency may even get magnified by the challenges of yoga asana practice. My personal experience is that the physical practice of hatha yoga alone is not strong enough medicine to change those patterns in today's world.

My dissatisfaction with yoga left me very aware of a longing for something more, a sad empty feeling. Remembering that my dad's prescription for the blahs was to do something helpful for someone else, I began to search for a way to take the focus off myself and still be myself. I had read about maitri, the loving-kindness aspect of Tibetan Buddhism, and was drawn to explore that, so when a friend of mine invited me to attend teachings with His Holiness the

Dalai Lama, I went. It was a two-week intensive retreat and the first week was slow going, with translators explaining to us Westerners the teachings of these great lamas. Some of the teachers wore business suits, some wore elaborate robes and exotic hairdos. I didn't have a clue who they were or what they were saying, but I liked being there. The second week His Holiness explained what it meant to be a bodhisattva—a person who dedicates their life to helping others—and without hesitation I signed on with a bodhisattva vow.

In the lobby I was surprised to find out that another friend, Rudy Wurlitzer, was there and that he was a longtime student of Buddhism. I was grateful when he took me under his wing and started taking me to teachings around town. All along he kept saying, "I think Gehlek Rimpoche is the teacher for you, but I don't know when he will be in New York City." One night shortly after that I was visiting my friend Philip Glass and just before I left he wrote me a little memo on the back of a piece of paper and folded it up. I didn't know that Phil was a student of Gehlek Rimpoche's but when I got home and opened the memo I discovered that it was written on the back of a notice announcing Gehlek Rimpoche's next teaching in New York. I called Phil and said, "Do you think it would be okay if I went to this?" and he said, "I think it means you're supposed to go!" Of course, I went and when I introduced myself to Rimpoche he seemed to already know my name. I had found my teacher.

BUDDHISM

Rimpoche taught me the basic premise of Buddhism—that life is suffering—and the practices of Buddhism, which ultimately lead us outward, rather than only inward. We start by sitting still and stabilizing our mind. From the spaciousness that arises during this practice of calm abiding, we naturally begin to feel our heart. Buddhism then offers us loving-kindness exercises that cultivate habits of compassion for ourselves and others. By staying with our feelings in an alert, nonjudgmental way, we begin to gain the courage to attend to our own tender heart by accepting who we are, warts and all. As this friendship with ourselves develops into a good habit, we begin to recognize other people's hearts, too, and feel inspired to be kind to them as well. We now have the ingredients of nongrasping wakefulness, compassion, benevolent energy, and disciplined power that make up the recipe for interacting intelligently, soulfully and spontaneously with ourselves, each other, our family, and the world.

These teachings invite us to open up to who we already are, rather than looking elsewhere for connection, because the seed of awakened heart is within all of us already: it's our heritage as human beings. It's just that we can't always feel our beautiful lotus heart blooming because we get stuck on ideas of fear, jealousy, anger, hatred, and greed.

Buddhist meditation techniques reveal that none of these emotions are solid, and with practice we learn how to watch them arise and fade away and still stay steady on our seat or on our feet. We learn how to remain in the immediacy of everything, to keep our awareness on doing our backbending, for example, rather than on what we are thinking about backbending. Then loving-kindness invites us to approach our backbends with at least an inner smile and a little less crabbiness.

Curiosity about what's really happening begins to rule over fear that our pleasure agenda will not get met. Not being attached to the outcome of our actions, but being more interested in experiencing our life at the same time that it's happening, opens us to the possibility of experiencing equanimity. Balance of body and mind, heart and mind, inner vision and outer awareness, giving and receiving, staying steady while riding the energy of our world.

After going on several retreats, reading dharma books, and meditating, I started to understand a little bit more about Buddhism. Mostly I noticed that it helped me in my life. I became more grounded, more patient, and more conscious of others. Over time, with the encouragement of my teacher, I began to share what I learned from him with my yoga students. The teachings and techniques were a natural fit with yoga asana practice.

Applying meditation instruction to yoga postures slowed me down enough to feel my breath, my heart, and my mind. Rather than looking for bliss by dropping out, I dropped in, taking notice of my physical sensations and the thoughts that arose in connection to them. I realized I had the same thought every time the teacher said, "Let's do backbending." I used to think I didn't like backbends, but my relationship to backbends changed when I simply recognized that thinking pattern. Letting go of that habit allowed my sense organs to soften and I began to experience each individual new backbend. I discovered that my backbends were different all the time and that was very interesting to me. In fact, I had been given license to be completely fascinated with my favorite subject—me—instead of trying to stifle my thoughts, repress my senses, and be different.

Yet I was confused when my meditation teachers said mindfulness meditation was "synchronizing body and mind." I understood that conceptually, but after sitting on the cushion for a whole weekend I thought, "What body?" Didn't the Buddha ever walk, stand, or climb stairs?

YOGA

History tells us that the Buddha did engage in extreme yogic practices—fasting, sleep deprivation, lengthy breath retention, standing on one leg for hours—and ultimately found them unsatisfactory. He discovered that trying to escape from your body and your world actually just generated more craving. Pretending that he didn't have a body or that it was a bad thing was equal to indulging in the body's desires. Ignoring the body doesn't work either because as long as you are inside a body, it will continue to try to get your attention one way or another. In an effort to escape desire he and his yoga buddies had locked out the possibility of any genuine feelings. Their fear of desire had eradicated all potential for happiness because who can feel joyful when their body is sick and wasting away?

When the Buddha recognized this, he realized that it was possible to replace denial with acceptance, to open up to the true nature of human experience, and to replace punishing asceticism with compassion. To the dismay of his yogi friends, he began moving toward a balanced state of health by eating some rice pudding. This action triggered the intriguing notion of middle ground: not too tight and not too loose.

Then he sat down under a tree and waited and watched. Many things happened while he sat under the tree. Beautiful, sexy women tried to seduce him. An army came from out of nowhere and shot arrows at him. Nature attacked him personally with storms that rained only over him. All these things happened, but just in his mind. He finally understood that and this realization woke him up. *Bodhi*—Buddha—means awake.

The mindfulness practice led him to observe his own thoughts and how they constantly fluctuate: feelings morph into other feelings and this is completely natural. Neither bad nor good. Then by applying compassion to this practice of paying attention (while doing yoga!) the Buddha found he could use his body as a vehicle not just for cutting through mental desire and craving but also for cultivating helpful states such as being kind, truthful, and content.

After forty nights under the tree he got up and began to move through the world again. (I wonder if he ever again felt like doing downward-facing dog pose after such a long meditation session.)

Patanjali is credited with writing his Yoga Sutra about 150 years later. Although yoga is often associated with Hinduism, it is most closely aligned with Sankhya, one of the six classical Indian darsanas, or "ways to see." Sankhya is an attempt to explain the nature of all existence by dividing it into Purusha, that which is unchanging, and Prakriti, or matter. It tells us that the separation of these two states is the cause of our suffering and that the path to liberation is through repression of our thoughts, withdrawal of our senses, and control of our body in order to reconnect with our true Self. Sankhya calls this union (this *re*-union) the state of yoga.

The practices of introverted concentration associated with this state are described in the Yoga Sutra of Patanjali as an eight-limbed path: yamas (restraints), niyamas (observances), asana (postures), pranayama (breathing), pratyahara (withdrawal of senses), dharana (concentration), dhyana (meditation), and samadhi (absorption). The limbs begin by refining our behavior in the outer world, then lead us more and more inward until we reach samadhi. Most people doing yoga today are engaged in the third limb, asana, which is a program of physical postures designed to purify the body and provide the physical strength and stamina required for long periods of immobility.

ASANA

The word *yoga* comes from the Sanskrit *yuj,* which means to yoke or bind, and is often translated as "union." In order to have union there must be at least two things coming together to become one, so yoga is another way of saying relationship. Nothing exists on its own and yoga reminds us of this through the physical practice of asana.

The word *hatha* means willful or forceful. Hatha yoga refers to a set of physically engaging exercises designed to align your skin, muscles, and bones. The asanas, or poses, are a system for reorganizing your physical architecture so that the drainpipe of your body becomes unclogged. This process opens the channels for your breath and energy to flow freely and for your neurological patterns to get remapped, soothed, and strengthened. When this kind of balance occurs, your body begins to feel even all over. This equanimity of sensation is a support and container for relaxed awareness in the mind and heart.

But who can say which should come first—a balanced body or a spacious mind? The reality is that each is elusive—more a process than a product, an experience rather than a commodity. Both process and experience imply a situation that is mobile, fluid, and engaging.

Asana practice offers us physical techniques for walking this balance beam between ease and steadiness. The word *asana,* often translated as "ground" or "seat," refers to the part of the body that is connected to the earth. Asana can also mean "to sit with." Being in the middle of what is happening within and without you can be explored through asana practice and in this way we begin to see how our body reflects our mind.

The process is similar to that in meditation: we place our bodies in various shapes and then "sit with" what comes up. Just like meditation practice, rather than applying an agenda right from the start, we are invited to take an unbiased approach toward what we observe. From our own intelligence, we then can make skillful decisions about how to work with our body using the means of balanced awareness, alignment, and effort.

AWAKENED UNION

At OM Yoga Center we practice a form of yoga called vinyasa, which is a series of flowing movement sequences coordinated with rhythmic breathing. We approach the vinyasa style with great attention to detail, especially regarding alignment, to ensure that students do not get injured and that they get the most benefit out of their practice. An equal element of OM yoga is meditation-in-action, which invites the yogi to observe and become familiar with mental and physical habits, to relax the grip of thought activity, and to kindly abide in the asana. All this while maintaining a sense of vipassana, or clear seeing, which opens the yogi to the world around him or her, creating a healthy balance to the refined inner vision of yoga practice. The flow, precision, and mindfulness of our yoga practice are all supported by Buddhist principles.

All of these exercises sit on a soft philosophical bed called ahimsa (non-harming) of yoga and maitri (loving-kindness) of Buddhism. What's the good of being awake if you can't let your heart be like your lungs, giving and receiving with every pulse? Mindfulness helps us recognize when we have habits that are harsh and creates a gap between that impulse and the action that usually follows. It creates a space for us to dip into our hearts and come back up with a pearl of kindness.

This is extremely helpful for yoga practitioners. Since for most of us a major part of our self-identity is tied to the appearance and health of our physicality, our body is an excellent reflective surface for getting to know our habits and applying ahimsa and maitri to what comes up. In the wordless conversation between our body and our mind, everything that happens in all our relationships—frustration, aggression, love, tenderness, boredom—will arise while doing a basic pose such as downward-facing dog. Yoga and meditation help us recognize our habitual form of effort—too tight or too loose—and naturally lead to a sensitivity regarding the actions of our body, speech, and mind. This is called right action, and it is made up of rhythm, movement, direction, energy, and intention, but never aggression.

When you apply this mind/heart training to the process of doing yoga asanas it becomes a way to understand the whole world in the form of you. It provides the means for working with all of those relationships right there on the yoga mat at the same time that you get more fit. And for us busy people who are both meditators and yogis as well as being moms, CEOs, and joggers, it is helpful to be able to combine practices.

Yoga helps Buddhists embody their meditation. As the meditator's body becomes more mobile, strong, and functional, it becomes a support for meditation practice rather than the more familiar and painful distraction of creaking knees and whining spines. Similarly, the specific focus of Buddhist mindfulness and compassion helps the yogi's mind become unbiased, wakeful, and connected in whatever physical shape he or she assumes and demonstrates the transient nature of all things, including mastery over body.

Sitting cross-legged at the end of yoga class, I feel elemental. My breath is the wind and my mind is a raft floating on the oceanic tide of prana. The fire in my belly radiates out and makes the sweat on my skin feel like rain and earth mixed together. My heart rests in a big, big space.

Then I get up off the mat and go back to running the yoga center. Hopefully, today I won't have a life-threatening experience, but still I'm grateful for my practices. Life might not be a bliss cloud, but through the wisdom and compassion of yoga and Buddhism, it has become supremely workable.

TWO
CALM ABIDING
How to Meditate

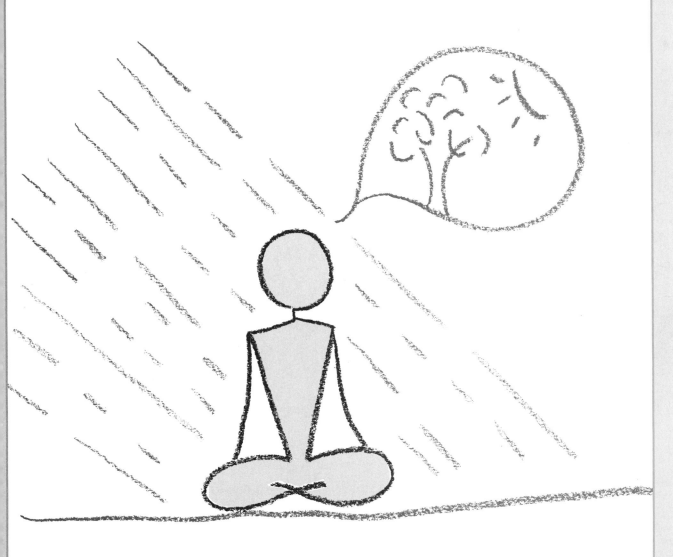

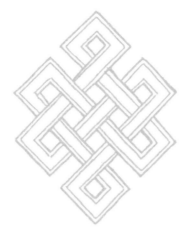

Buddha Mind

Lately I've been feeling a tad guilty when I teach yoga to beginners. Especially if they have traveled from a cold place and a stressful job to a beautiful, warm retreat in the Caribbean. Even more so if they were tempted by one of those pictures of a healthy, radiant yogini on the beach looking oh! so blissful and serene.

I'm going to reveal one of the best-kept secrets of the world: practicing yoga is not the same thing as relaxing. I realize that the people who come to retreats looking for a siesta-like yoga experience may be disappointed, but turning your body upside down and inside out and then staying there for even three or four breaths is simply not a piece of cake. Not to mention untying yourself from pretzel-like positions. What they are really looking for is a perfect breeze swaying the big, cozy hammock they're snoozing in with the soothing background accompaniment of soft waves rolling on the shore. That's relaxing.

The experience of yoga asana practice can be one of more spaciousness in the body, but that takes time and patience. Unless that yogini on the beach is practicing with a conscious sense of mindfulness and ease, as soon as her back starts to feel tight, the external comfort—beach, sky, water—will vanish as her entire inner experience becomes all about her discomfort.

It turns out that the answer is not in changing the external environments in which we find ourselves, but in understanding the internal environment of our own mind. It has been said that our mind is like the weather—it changes all the time and we can never get away from it. No matter where we go and no matter what the weather is like outside, it is our mind that determines whether we feel stormy or breezy, cold or warm, relaxed or claustrophobic.

How can we learn not to get so easily shaken by external phenomena? How can we learn to remain composed within life's ups and downs? How can yoga help us find a sense of comfort within any situation? How can our yoga be a practice for living? It all depends on your point of view.

The story of Shakyamuni Buddha is a good example of this. Raised as a prince in a beautiful palace with every possible luxury—food, entertainment, education, servants, a loving wife and child—he found himself discontent with his situation and curious about the bigger world outside. His father had given strict orders to the palace guards to never let his son leave the palatial compound, but one night, he managed to slip out. On that night he saw for the first time a sick person, an old person, and a dead person, and he understood that what he saw in those people would happen to him and to everyone else in the entire world.

He was struck by the fact that everything changes and he had a great realization that his perfect world would not last forever. When he returned to the palace this knowledge made it impossible for him to be comfortable within the confines of a false universe because he knew that even that would change. So he left the palace again in the middle of the night and began his search for deeper understanding through the practices of yoga and meditation. He eventually shared his discoveries in the form of teachings that over the centuries have come to be called Buddhism, beginning with the Four Noble Truths.

Buddhism teaches us the truth of impermanence—the fact that everything changes. We can get blown about by change, or we can learn to ride change. Sometimes change is so slow that we can miss it and remain stuck in our comfortable—but sleepy—habits. Sometimes change is so fast that we get scared and overreact with too much energy, or—the opposite—become paralyzed.

Relating to change in these ways is not uncommon. The Buddha outlined this in the First and Second Noble Truths. The First Noble Truth is that suffering exists. If we only relate to change by denying it or getting upset we will miss out on life or be unhappy much of the time.

The Second Noble Truth is that we create our own suffering. In Buddhist philosophy the cause of suffering is not what arises in our life, but our attitude toward it—how we tend to want situations or people to be different than they are, to go away or to remain forever, or to change in exactly the way we want.

Since change is inevitable, it is to our benefit to develop skillful means to stay awake when change is rolling slow like the muddy Mississippi and to relax and hold on when life feels like a bucking bronco ride.

What are these skillful means and how can we develop them? The Third Noble Truth says we can be free from suffering and the Fourth Noble Truth tells us how to be free from suffering. One of the main elements on the path is right understanding, developed through the practice of mindfulness meditation, called shamatha, or calm abiding.

SHAMATHA

Shamatha practice is a technique for staying centered within our evolving world. It's not about creating an unmoving blissful state, but about having the

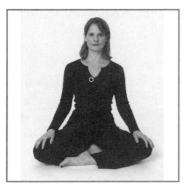

courage to experience all the states of mind that arise and pass, just like weather. It's a practice of waking up to what is happening around us and being in the middle of that right then and there. In other words, being in the present moment.

When we can begin to stop wishing things were different and learn to ride movement, we will shift toward a state of balance of unconditional contentment. This is called santosha, and it is one of the niyamas, or guiding principles, of yoga. This sense of balance, contentment, or equanimity naturally arises when you can stay in the middle of what's going on, without wishing it were different. Chögyam Trungpa, a renowned Buddhist teacher, used to say, "Lean into it." So instead of trying to avoid things—the hamstring stretch of downward-facing dog, the fear of inversions, the intimacy of relationships—we go in even deeper. A lot of bravery is required to open to the many varieties of richness that life offers. That's why we have to practice it.

Here's how you do shamatha.

TAKING YOUR SEAT

We begin by connecting back to the earth simply by sitting down on it. This is the first step toward relating to our reality rather than trying to transcend or escape to a different place.

But sitting on the floor with your legs crossed may be extremely uncomfortable. Although we have discussed that our practice is a way to become comfortable within uncomfortable situations, it doesn't mean that once you have seen clearly where you are, you shouldn't work with your environment to create a supportive situation. In other words, accessorize.

You may wish to place a cushion or two under your seat, which will allow your hips to open and your spine to lift. Close your eyes. Snuggle your sitting bones down, firmly grounding your seat on the cushion. Turn your palms down on your thighs just above your knees. This hand position, or mudra, is called "resting the mind" and you may feel how it puts a soft lid on any kind of over-stimulated energy you may be experiencing.

Feel the weight of your arms resting on your thighs, inviting your legs and pelvis to drop earthward. See if you can find a corresponding lift in the chest, letting your heart feel light, bright, and buoyant.

With your mind's eye, begin to travel up the ladder of your spine, feeling as if you are growing up out of the ground. Let your ribs lift up off your pelvis. Allow your belly to be soft and relaxed. Your vertebrae actually go all the way up to between your ears, so try moving your head around a little bit and see if you can have a sensation of the skull balancing delicately on the top of your spine.

Relax your jaw and let your tongue drop down to the bottom of your mouth. Soften the inner corners of your eyes.

Feel the strong quality of the back of your body and let it give you confidence, a reminder of your own basic goodness. Feel the contrasting softness and vulnerability of the front of your body, letting that remind you to stay open to whatever arises.

Now slowly open your eyes and rest your vision on the floor about five feet in front of you. Keep your gaze soft and wide without going fuzzy. Think of your vision as being panoramic.

This is called taking your seat. The earth is our witness for all that we experience. It is our support and will never let us down. So we begin by taking our seat and reaffirming as our heritage the right to sit with humble confidence.

WATCHING YOUR BREATH

The way to stay in the center of your experience is to be in the present moment. Since most of us have wandering minds, we need a reference point, a landmark that will ground us firmly in the present moment, something that is always in the now. The most prevalent thing is our breath. Our breath is never in the past or future but always only happening right now, right here.

Begin to watch your breath moving out and moving in. Try not to change your breathing in any way. Just breathe naturally. Each time you exhale, let your mind soften and flow out on your breath and mix with the space all around you.

When you realize that you've gotten caught up in a thought, that's no problem at all. Simply note that activity by saying to yourself, "Thinking," and return your attention to your breath once again.

MEETING YOUR MIND

Sometimes we have a notion that meditation is going to be one thing—peaceful. But as soon as you sit down and get quiet you will undoubtedly notice that your mind is full of thoughts. One quiet Saturday morning during a weekend meditation retreat I startled myself by jolting awake out of a dense brain fog with the thought, "Oh, no, I'm going to get in trouble for making so much noise!" Then I looked around and quickly saw that I was in the meditation hall and hadn't been bothering anyone but myself! That's how thick and loud my mental activity was that morning.

Most of us have a constant inner soundscape similar to a James Joyce novel—no punctuation, no gaps, just a constant run-on sentence of gossip, plans, regrets, and songs from the radio. In fact, our minds are like this all the time but it's only when we still our physical activity that we begin to notice our mind activity. Gaining an awareness of the activity of the mind is at the heart of mindfulness meditation practice.

Like a chicken laying eggs, our mind generates thoughts. This is not considered to be a problem and meditation practice is not an attempt to change this. The process of repeatedly labeling thoughts—saying to ourselves, "Thinking," whenever we realize we're doing it—is a technique for helping us to increase our awareness of habitual mind activity and to let go of each thought as we become aware of it.

Please do not try to block out all your thoughts. Many people have the idea that meditation is about emptying your head, but having a blank mind has never been shown to be beneficial for human beings. A better meditation is not one with less thoughts, and a session with no thoughts is not the best. There is no good or bad here. The point is simply to wake up to the fact that we generally experience a wall of thoughts that can draw us away from our present experience.

Try not to discriminate between types of thoughts, only letting go of ugly thoughts and lingering on pleasant ones. Mindfulness meditation practice will lead you to a recognition of recurring thought patterns specific to you. No matter what the thought, without judging it in any way, once again gently say to yourself, "Thinking," and return your attention to the movement of your breath. This process of waking up and coming back to nowness will happen over and over.

This is practice for becoming familiar with how our own minds work. Well-known meditation teacher Pema Chödron calls this process "making friends with yourself."

TOUCH AND GO

When you notice a thought, touch it by feeling the texture of it. Is it aggressive, sad, frightening, boring, inspiring? Without repressing it, experience the sensuous element of the thought, let that feeling linger, and then let it go and return to the breathing.

For example, out of nowhere a memory may arise of Aunt Mabel's apple pie. You may experience this as a feeling of warmth, which you can drop into fully, then say to yourself, "Thinking," and return to your breathing. Without the technique of shamatha meditation, what might happen instead is that you have a thought of Aunt Mabel's apple pie, then you wish you could get up off the meditation cushion and go get a piece of pie from the bakery right now and then you remember that you don't have any money so you have to go to the bank and that's in the other direction and now you begin to debate whether you should take the car or just eat the ice cream that's in the refrigerator already but of course, wouldn't it be good to have both the ice cream and the apple pie but you promised yourself that you wouldn't eat any more desserts until your birthday, which you still haven't figured out how to celebrate this year. Sound familiar? This is called a story line and it often follows on the heels of the initial thought. It's clear that this will take you away from sensory experience and launch you fully into the past or future. Of course, when that happens, it's fine. As soon as you notice it, with no judgment, once again just label it thinking.

Seeing thoughts as they arise, tasting them, labeling them, and returning to the breath again and again is the technique for beginning to recognize that we all have many thoughts, often recurring ones, but that none of them are solid. If we stay steady on our seat, we will see that all thoughts, happy and sad, simply float up to the surface and then fade away. We can go through as many experiences on the meditation cushion as off and that's why this is called practice.

PATH WITHOUT A GOAL

Now you have learned the technique of shamatha, or calm abiding: taking your seat, watching your breath, meeting your mind, and touch and go. But if good thoughts are not cherished over bad thoughts and there is no value attached to a blank mind, what's the goal? How can you tell if you're getting anywhere?

Meditation practice is a challenge for many of us simply because of that question. Try not to approach this with a project mentality. In fact, this is an opportunity to let go of the habit of managing things, organizing your life, checking things off your list, and getting on with it. Meditation is not a task-oriented activity. In fact, it is only slightly an activity. It is just as much about receptivity.

So the final instruction is to place only 25 percent of your attention on your breath. Let your awareness of your mind extend out to your environment. Don't try to shut out sounds, smells, or your world in any way.

While leading a meditation session, yoga teacher Erich Schiffmann once said that although it seems like it would be the opposite, expanding is never egotistical but shrinking is. Let your meditation be a process of opening to your own mind, to your feelings, to what the world offers you. Without judging anything or wishing it were different, this process can lead to an expansion of who you think you are and what you think you can contain.

FRESH STARTS

Oftentimes when new meditators begin they become frustrated because they feel they can't catch every thought as it arises. Other people sit for thirty years before they remember to use the technique of mentally noting "thinking."

There is a middle way between these two, which is more an attitude than an actual measure of how you're doing. Try not to get supervigilant with corralling in your stampeding mind cattle and at the same time don't space out, losing awareness altogether until your butt falls asleep and wakes up your mind.

When you realize that you've spaced out, refresh your posture and take a fresh start with the whole thing. No problem.

When you realize that you are giving yourself a headache because you are concentrating so hard on what's going on in there, let go of the technique, close your eyes, take a few deep breaths, reorganize your posture, and begin again. No problem—because this is a process you can never finish, and you can always begin again.

Special Tips

- Creating the proper environment is important. Although we are not trying to shut out the world, it is still a good idea to set some boundaries for your practice. Make sure you turn on your answering machine and turn off your cell phone.

- Choose a period of time for your sitting meditation practice and stick to it. Thirty minutes is a good length to begin. Even if you end up playing with your toenails, stay there for the duration. Eventually this discipline will transform into a powerful friend.

- Try to practice on a regular basis but don't punish yourself if you don't. Once a week is okay and once a day is okay. Figure out what works in your schedule and make it realistic. Find the middle path between holding a rigid commitment and being lazy.

- You may also begin to experience physical discomfort—aching back, whining hips, sleeping legs. It is fine to shift your posture if your physical pain is too much. When you move, you still follow the technique of watching the breath and labeling your thoughts "Thinking." Make sure that when you move it is because you really need to and not just because you are bored and restless.

Remember there is a difference between practice and perfection. Meditation is only something you can practice. At the same time that you can never do it perfectly you can always do it perfectly as long as your intention is openhearted.

After you've been meditating for a while you'll discover that, just like everything else in life, your sitting practice may be uplifting, challenging, boring, ordinary, weird, joyous, or magical. Possibly all of the above, in only thirty minutes.

What we are practicing is not to change any of that, but to sit still while the movie of our mind plays out. Noticing when we get caught up in a particular scene or dialogue and coming back to the present moment, over and over again.

Let your meditation be a practice of awakening and connecting with all that is. It's deep but it doesn't have to be heavy. Remember, you're just sitting still, watching the movie of your own mind. Try to stay relaxed and see if you can approach your own practice with a healthy combination of mindfulness, playfulness, precision, and curiosity.

THREE

THE INVISIBLE BRIDGE

How to Breathe

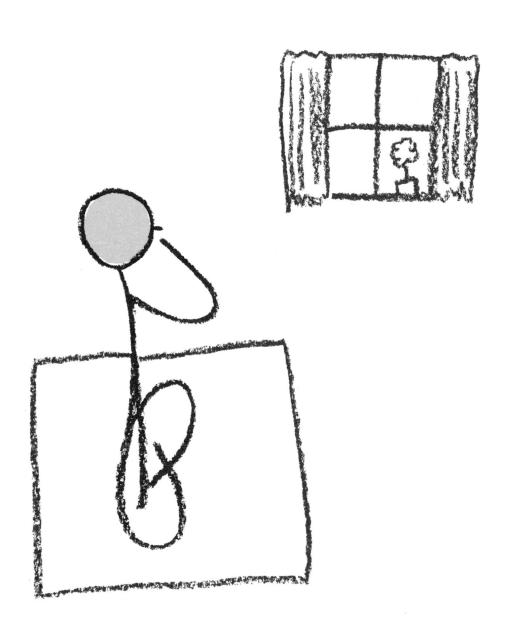

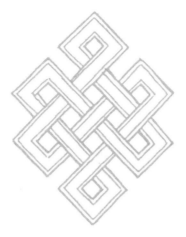

Yoga Body

Downtown Manhattan has been my home for over twenty years. My apartment was not affected as badly as many others, but for about two months following September 11, my husband and I could smell the fires. It was particularly intense in the first weeks after the attacks. During that period, I kept waking up in the middle of the night. I slowly came to realize that the smoky air was waking me up because unconsciously, I didn't want to take it into my body. Throughout the city there was talk about air safety concerns and this united us. But there was another level of concern that slowly surfaced in our consciousness. People began to delicately talk about how the smoke was coming from the remains of our fellow New Yorkers who had lost their lives. This was an intense visceral relationship with those people with whom we all felt so heart-connected, and the powerful experience of our breathing alone was our primary method of acknowledging and continuing this exchange, this giving and receiving of life in various forms.

Paying attention to our breathing is the most immediate way to remind us of our connection to all of nature, including human nature. The organic rhythm of the breath itself relates to the entire universe: everything in nature vibrates, pulsates, expands, and contracts constantly, even things that appear solid, like floors and rocks. They are just vibrating at a slower rhythm.

Since the breath connects our outer world and our inner world, the more we become aware of our breath, the more we begin to dissolve the boundary between these two worlds, and between ourselves and others. Breath is a constant exchange with others—we all breathe the same air. It has been said that the air we breathe today will be breathed by someone on the opposite side of the world tomorrow.

Even just the slightest hint of breath awareness can begin to change your life—when you get tense, are stuck in traffic, receive an unexpected letter from the IRS—you might notice that your breath changes. Usually it gets quicker and more shallow or stops altogether for a few tense moments. Once you learn to recognize your own form of habitual breathing response, you have the opportunity to consciously rebalance your inhalation and exhalation. This rebalancing will pacify your nervous system and change your relationship to whatever upset you in the first place. Rather than allowing our response to an event affect our breathing, we can learn instead to let our breathing change our relationship to the event. The breath is the invisible bridge between our mind and our body.

In our meditation practice we place about 25 percent of our attention on our breath. This technique uses the breath as a primary object or home base for being "in-body." But meditation is not about the breath. It is about watching our mind. We simply use the breath as a landmark of the present moment, because the breath is never in the past or present, but always happening right here and now.

This is different from yogic breathing exercises in which we learn to focus our attention on the movement of the breath as a method of developing a personal understanding of our own physical and energetic connection of body and mind. This is called breath awareness and it allows us to see where the circulation of wind energy in our body is blocked and where it is free. With this information, we can make intelligent choices about how we want to manipulate the breath in various ways that soothe our nervous system, cleanse our sinuses, and oxygenate our entire body, leading to a sense of well-being and harmonious rejuvenation.

PRANAYAMA

We are always breathing. Yet, just like waves on the shore, like snowflakes and fingerprints, each breath is unique. But they all look alike unless you take a good look. The ancient yogis said that we are each given a certain number of these one-of-a-kind breaths per lifetime. If we extend each breath, we can extend our lifetime, so it's recommended that we breathe slowly and deeply, as well as pay close attention to our breathing. This is the only function of our body that is both voluntary and involuntary.

While we might not be able to watch every single breath, we can start the process by doing breath observation and breath manipulation exercises called pranayama, which means extension (*ayama*) of life force (*prana*). *Prana* is also translated to mean "to bring forth mystical vibration"—that ineffable energy that exists in sunlight, water, earth, plants, animals, people, and wind or breath.

For us humans, the most direct way to feel this universal life force is through the wavelike nature of our breathing. This reminds us that even though everything is changing all the time, we can still feel peaceful, as long as we keep in rhythm.

Whenever you feel out of sync, take a moment to lengthen and equalize your inhale and exhale. Right away you will feel more balanced. The act of mindfully watching our breathing can have just as profound an effect as watching the ocean waves—it can help us feel alive and expansive.

This is called taking a fresh start. It's available to us every moment! The only problem is that we forget about it. How can we develop the positive habit of taking a fresh start on a regular basis?

LOCATING THE BREATH

We can begin by introducing ourselves to our body's breathing anatomy. Try this:

Sit or lie down and touch the front of your bottom ribs. Trace the shape of your ribs around the sides and as far toward the back as you can reach. Then feel the second rib up from the bottom. Now explore the area between the bottom and second rib. This is a muscle called the intercostal, which allows the rib cage to open and close like a bellows as we inhale and exhale. Continue your investigation all the way to the top of your chest. Notice how your ribs are shaped, how they are like a ladder that goes under your armpits, how they go up your back all the way to your neck. Take time to feel how your ribs move more in some places than in others. Are there areas of your rib cage that seem tighter or more free? Are there places that are more or less sensitive? Can you direct your breath into the tight or dead spots?

Now that you have met your rib cage, lie down on your back with your knees bent and feet flat on the floor, wide apart, and pigeon-toed, so that your knees fall together naturally, allowing your thigh muscles to relax. Place your palms on your lower abdomen, below your navel. Breathe naturally and let your hands ride up and down on the tide of your breath, like a little raft floating on the ocean.

After a few minutes, move your hands up to your middle belly, just above your navel, including your bottom ribs. What does your breath feel like here? Is it tighter, more or less fluid? Do your hands feel heavy? Can you feel the movement of your diaphragm—dropping down with each inhale, and lifting up like an umbrella as you exhale? The diaphragm is a perfect example of cleaving—it both joins and separates the upper, more heavenly organs of the heart and lungs with the visceral, more earthly abdominal organs.

Finally, place your hands on your chest and let your breath move your hands here. Be curious about each of these areas: explore under the armpits, between each rib, right side versus left side. Can you feel your breath moving into the back of your body against the floor?

GUIDED BREATH AWARENESS EXERCISE

Sit in a comfortable cross-legged position. Sit on a cushion or two, elevating your hips as much as you need to in order to allow your spine to grow straight up out of the flowerpot of your pelvis. Find a vertical pelvis by letting the tailbone and pubic bone move toward each other. You will be sitting like this for about five minutes. If you want to sit against a wall, put a small pillow at the base of your spine so you can sit upright without leaning back.

Feel free to touch your ribs, belly, or chest anytime during these exercises. Imagine you have nostrils in the tight places and breathe deeply there.

Close your eyes and notice the movement of your breath. Make sure you are breathing both in and out through the nose. Isn't it interesting that even though you don't consciously change it, just by paying attention to the breath, it changes slightly?

Slowly begin to deepen the inhalation and extend the exhalation. Don't go to your very deepest inhale right away. Go slowly, getting deeper and fuller, little by little, breath by breath. Notice how the breath moves the ribs, which warms up the intercostal muscles and how that, in turn, allows the breath to deepen. Keep watching.

Now feel how the inhalation drops down into your body. Let it descend all the way to your groins, the hollows at the junction of your legs and pelvis. Then, like water in a glass, feel the breath begin to fill your torso all the way up to your collarbones.

Let the exhale begin from the bottom as well. Even though you know your breath is coming up and out of your nose, imagine that you are exhaling out of your heart. Feel how this heart-exhale creates spaciousness in the chest and possibly feelings of lightness, joy, and bravery.

Again, like a waterfall, let the inhalation flow all the way down to your groins and slowly fill you up to the top. As you exhale, let the breath rise up like a fountain issuing out of your open heart.

Tie your mind to your breath. When you notice that you've spaced out, take a fresh start. Try to take deep, full breaths without tightening at the top of the inhale or hardening at the bottom of the exhale. If that happens, don't worry about it. It can take many years of practice before the breath becomes free and even.

Repeat as many times as you like.

CALMING BREATH

The calming breath is called sama vritti, which means equal fluctuation. Breathing in and out for the same length of time is the best way to calm your nervous system and, in turn, your mind.

Sit in a comfortable cross-legged position. Exhale completely. Inhale for five counts. Exhale for five counts. If this is too long or too short, change it to a length that is comfortable for you today. Repeat as many times as you like.

ALTERNATE NOSTRIL CALMING BREATH

Alternate nostril calming breath is called surya chandra sama vritti, which means "sun moon equal fluctuation." In yoga the left side of the body relates

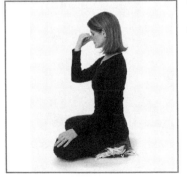

to the moon and is considered cooling, receptive, and feminine. The right side of the body is the sun—heating, active, and masculine. Breathing through alternate nostrils is one method for creating balance in these two aspects of our energy. It is said that the nostrils naturally alternate between being more or less open. When one is open the other one is at least partially blocked. There is a brief moment in between when they are both open and we experience balance naturally. Otherwise you may feel more practical sometimes, and at other times more poetic.

Make the hand signal for OK with your left hand by joining the thumb and index fingertips; this is called jnana, or wisdom, mudra. A mudra is a seal, or circle of energy. With your right hand, make vishnu mudra, placing the first two fingers—index and middle fingers—in the palm of your hand. Join your baby finger to your ring finger, and bring this mudra up to your nose. Make sure you are not dropping your nose down to meet your finger, but lifting your hand up to meet your nose. Lift your wrist slightly to place your thumb on the shelf of your right nostril and your ring finger on the shelf of your left nostril.

Alternately close and open each nostril to allow the breath in and out. Be very gentle with your nose as you do this exercise. Try not to squish it from side to side.

Begin by exhaling completely. Close your right nostril and inhale left for five counts. Close the left nostril. Lift your thumb and exhale out of your right nostril for five counts. Then inhale through the right nostril for five counts. Block the right nostril and lift your ring finger. Exhale out of the left nostril for five counts.

Begin again. Repeat the entire sequence at least three times.

NOT TOO TIGHT, NOT TOO LOOSE

One day, a musician was playing a stringed instrument. He asked the Buddha, "How should I meditate?"

The Buddha said, "How do you tune your instrument?"

The musician said, "Not too tight, not too loose."

The Buddha replied, "Exactly like that."

How should we use our breathing in our asana practice? As in meditation practice, your attention is placed on the movement of the breath to keep your mind in your body. But you can also deepen your breathing pattern, as in the calming breath technique.

Paying attention to the sound and texture of your breath during your asana practice gives you instant feedback on the quality of your practice in each moment. Just as we don't want our mind to get too narrowly focused or too widely divergent, and we don't want to grip our muscles or relax them altogether, we want our breath to flow with a balance of voluntary and involuntary force.

We already know that asana practice can be vigorous, so we use our breath as part of the way we discover balance, stability, and equanimity within challenging situations. If the breath gets too harsh, hard, or loud, you will be making a stressful situation even more so. Overly effortful breathing can agitate your nervous system. The quality of your breath, your attention, and your physical activity should be in harmony with each other and in harmony with what you want to practice. Do you want to practice harshness, aggression, pushing, grasping, agitation? Of course not. Let your breath be a mirror of what you want to practice.

Think of your body as a tube and let the breath run through the middle of the tube without chafing along the edges. Listen to the sound of the breath. It should be only loud enough for you to hear it. Let your conscious breathing be like playing an instrument—not too tight, not too loose.

Many people think of yoga as just stretching. But if we only try to get bigger and go out, out, out, it would be like taking a huge breath in . . . and never exhaling. That's not stretching, that's grasping. Without a connection to the breath, yoga is just a series of frozen shapes that solidfy whatever opinions we already have about who we are and what our bodies can do.

With proper understanding and a little pranayama practice under your belt, the rhythm of breathing in and breathing out can be your guide as you begin to learn or deepen your yoga practice. Eventually it will become a seamless process of extending and gathering, of falling back to center and radiating out, over and over again. When we experience this natural sway in our body, mind, and breath, we begin to feel a connection to the changing seasons, the movement of night and day, the flow of the tides, and the heartbeat of all beings. We begin to make yoga—union—with everything and everybody. When we can do this we will begin to experience an even greater sense of balance between the three aspects of our being—body, breath, and mind.

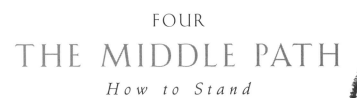

FOUR
THE MIDDLE PATH
How to Stand

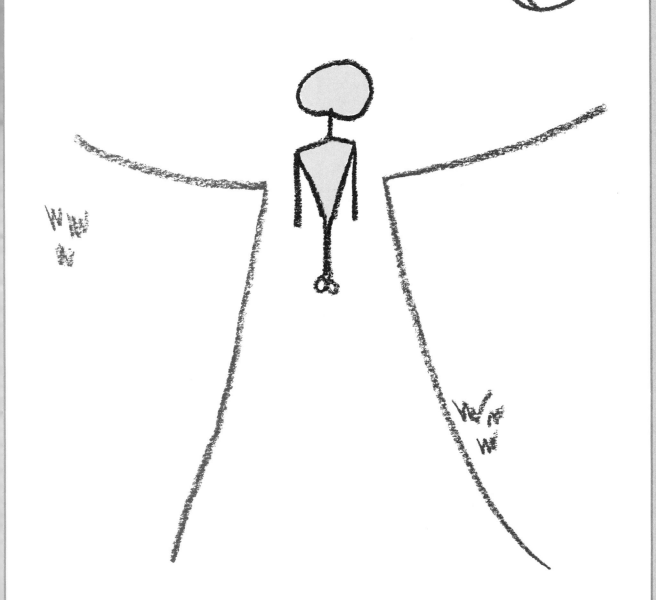

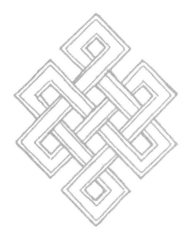

YOGA BODY

Not long ago my dad, a recent yoga convert full of curiosity about the practice, saw me sitting in sukhasana and asked, "What's the name of that pose?" When I told him it was called easy pose, his response was a snort followed by, "Easy for who?" Good question, Dad.

The Yoga Sutra of Patanjali says that yoga asanas should be practiced with steadiness and ease. The dictionary defines ease as freedom from pain, labor, discomfort, anxiety, or great effort; a quiet state of mind. But how can we feel any of those freedoms when we've got these big gross bodies that are stiff and tight and sore and weak and all the time getting chubbier?

It's all about perception. Even the official definitions of ease are divided equally between the physical and the mental, leaving "freedom from great effort" to fall into both categories.

Candace Pert, former chief brain biochemist for the National Institute of Mental Health, said, "In the end I find I can't separate brain from body. Consciousness isn't just in the head. Nor is it a question of mind over body. If one takes into account the DNA directing the dance of the peptides, [the] body is the outward manifestation of the mind."

In other words, our mind is everywhere in our body. The path to steadiness and ease is to consciously unite the two. At the same time that our yoga practice cultivates the physical stamina for meditation, we can purposefully take an approach of ease that will enable our physical experience to be one of opening, as well.

It's this notion of union that's at the heart of our hatha yoga and meditation practices. Science tells us that every cell in our body has the same qualities as a whole person—respiration, elimination, pulsation—so we know conceptually that there is conciousness in every nook and cranny of our physical being. The problem is that we have not cultivated the habit of experiencing or relating to our mind and body as interconnected. You may even forget you have a body until it gets hungry or too big for your clothes or overcooked by the sun. We feed it, clothe it, bathe it, and share it with certain people, but otherwise tend to relate to our body as the downstairs neighbor that is inferior to the talking head who lives upstairs.

Often we experience our own body as an external environment that we inhabit. If we are learning through meditation practice that we can stay centered within changing environments and situations, it could be said that our body is the most immediate external environment we know. And just like all external environments, our body is changing all the time. Many of us wish it would change in different ways than it is going on its own! Most people wish they were thinner or taller or had longer legs or bigger breasts or something that they can't control. As you grow older, you tend to wish for a stronger body, a more reliable body, good digestion, elastic skin, and enough hair to cover the top of your head. Even our desire for what we want in our body changes. How can we ever find a place of relaxation, of acceptance, of ease and at the same time work in ways that will cultivate the physical confidence and steadiness that arises from skeletal strength, muscular flexibility, and organic health? It's all about taking the middle path.

Throughout our practice, and this book, we will explore the dynamic relationship between up and down, out and in, active and receptive, masculine and feminine, effort and release, flow and structure, form and space. We can begin our study with the foundation of all the asanas, tadasana.

TADASANA

Tadasana is also called mountain pose and just like a mountain it joins heaven and earth. The principles of tadasana are a primer for learning how to do the Four Noble Actions—standing, walking, sitting, and lying down—with strength, confidence, and grace. The alignment, action, rotation, and coordination techniques for manifesting balance in tadasana are the foundation for every other yoga pose.

JOINING HEAVEN AND EARTH

Begin by standing with your feet together, toes and heels touching. If you are a beginner, if you have balance issues, or if the shape or size of your legs makes it difficult to bring your feet together, then place your feet directly below your sitting bones.

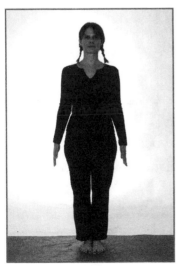

In tadasana, the asana, or seat of the pose, is your feet. In order to establish a strong connection to the earth, lift your feet up one at a time and stamp them down. Feel the quality of the ground's support underneath you. Feel the texture of the floor under the skin of your feet.

Now bend over and press the top of your big toe ball joint with your thumb and the baby toe ball joint with your index finger. Next touch the inner, and then the outer, heels of each foot. These four points are called the four corners of the foot. Work

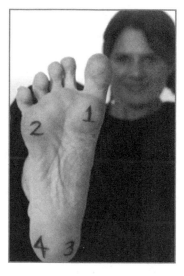

on maintaining balance in the middle of these points, which will be approximately the front of your heel or where a spat would be on old-fashioned shoes.

Stand up again and, keeping the four corners of the feet grounded, lift just your toes up off the floor and fan them wide apart. See if you can maintain the space between each toe as you lower them back to the floor one by one, beginning with the baby toe. Become familiar with your own personal toes. Which ones are in love with each other and never want to separate? Which ones require a lot of effort to move together? Can you feel the wind between your toes? Do you notice any relationship between those observations and your shoes—stilettos, flip-flops, sneakers? Feel free to use your more dexterous fingers to create an equal amount of space between each toe.

Just as in meditation, when you are invited to simply see what is what, continue to explore your body with curiosity and nonjudgment. Whatever you learn about yourself is the first step toward recognizing your patterns of movement and how your yoga practice might be able to help you create more balance in your body.

Moving up the body, place your hands on your hips and feel the bony quality of your pelvis. Is one hip higher than the other?

Place your hands on the middle of your chest and feel your heart beating. What other movements can you feel here?

Touch the top of your head and feel the weight of your hands there.

Keep one hand on your head and place the other hand on your sacrum. Feel the relationship between the two bones.

Keep your hand on your sacrum and place the other one over your heart. What do you feel here?

Keep your hand on your heart and place the other one on the top of your head. Who is the boss today—your head or your heart?

Now extend both arms sideways out from your shoulders. Reach through every single fingertip as you slowly lower your arms down by your sides.

Reconnect your feet earthward and extend upward through the top of your head. Maintain this sense of expansive energy in all directions.

Let your tongue drop to the bottom of your mouth and relax your jaw—ahhhh. Slightly lift the corners of your mouth. Feel the roof of the mouth open and imagine that opening extending all the way through the crown of your head.

Feel the front of your face softening and falling toward the back of your head.

Let your eyes rest in the middle of the sockets. Keep them open and see what is right in front of you. Can you soften your eyes and still stay focused so that you can take in what it is that you are looking at?

Feel your breath. Feel the light around you. Notice the taste of your mouth. Hear all the sounds around you.

Synchronizing down and up, right and left, front and back, are all physical manifestations of joining heaven and earth. Heaven represents our vision or aspirations, and earth is the action required to make the dreams happen. The heaven aspect relates to creativity and vision but can be expressed as a head-in-the-clouds dreamer. The earth aspect is a grounded quality that shows up as getting things done, but with a plodding nature that never steps out of the box. The potential for combining the two lies solely in the domain of human beings.

Tadasana is the reference point for all other poses because it establishes our physical alignment. But it also helps us to deepen our understanding of the alignment between body and mind, the middle path between intention and action.

Standing in tadasana is a reminder that the yogic middle path means never going only to the left, only up, or only forward. In yoga we always move in more than one direction at the same time. To extend up, we drop down. To radiate out, we connect to our center. To reach through our fingertips, we plug our arms into our shoulder joints. To see and hear more vividly, we soften our eyes and our ears.

Tadasana appears to be a simple static pose, but on deeper investigation we discover that it is very alive. Just like a mountain there are flowing and obstructed rivers of energy, fluids, and wind. There are relationships created by the topography of our bodyscape. There are slow, subtle movements that take patience to observe. The mountain pose body and the mountain pose mind become mirrors of each other just like a mountain sees itself reflected in a lake.

MASCULINE AND FEMININE COORDINATION
PELVIS AND LEGS

In addition to willful or forceful, the word *hatha* is also translated as *ha,* which means sun, and *tha,* which means moon. In yoga philosophy, the sun holds the qualities of heat and activity, which relate to the masculine aspect in all of us. The moon is the feminine aspect that expresses our cool, receptive nature. For all

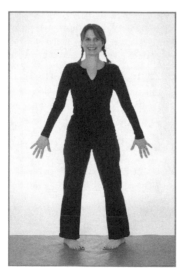

of us to be whole, we need to familiarize ourselves with both sides of this equation and begin to develop a healthy bonding between the two.

Let's explore this relationship in our pelvis and shoulders, the two most powerful areas for expression and receptivity. Both the legs and arms can roll in and out. Lie down on your back and play around with this a little bit and notice what happens in your chest and pelvis. When the arms and legs roll in toward the body, our energy draws inward and becomes quiet or possibly repressed. This is called internal rotation.

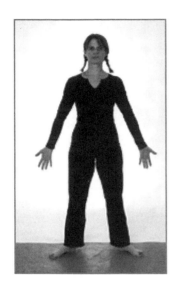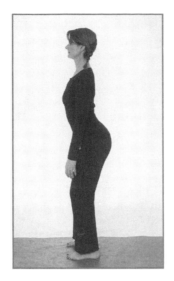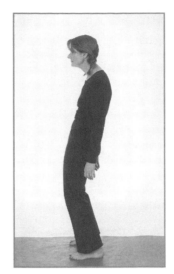

When the arms and legs roll out, we have more physical freedom but we may feel overexposed. Our energy is expressed in an outgoing flow. This is called external rotation.

We need both internal and external rotation in every position in order to find the middle path in our skeletal alignment and eventually our energy body.

Stand in tadasana and try this exercise to begin getting a sense of balance in your pelvis. Let your knees soften and turn in so you become pigeon-toed. Tip your pelvis to spin your buttocks upward. This is called internal rotation of the legs. This relates to the feminine aspect of our energy, which is very light and airy. This internal rotation spins the pubic bone back between the thighs and deepens the groins, which allows breath and prana to flow into the pelvic floor and creates space for movement in the joint.

But without the element of external rotation it is only half the picture. Now try the reverse. Tuck your pelvis way under and let your knees and toes point out. This is considered the masculine aspect, which is earthly but without some imagination could become the kind of downward-moving energy that you could get stuck in—like quicksand.

To unite the feminine and masculine in your pelvis, return your pelvis back to the internal rotation tilt. Try to maintain the depth in the groins as you slowly draw your tailbone forward to meet the pubic bone, bringing your inner thighs and heels together. Now you should feel that your legs are in parallel alignment with each other, toes pointing straight ahead, weight balanced on the four corners of the feet. As the pubic bone and tailbone move together, this creates a dynamic toning in the pelvic floor, an uplifted energy, which is a good support for the earthy abdominal organs.

The balance of internal and external rotation creates neutral, or what we call parallel, alignment. Each of us will need a different percentage of inward and outward to get to the middle. It depends on where you start. If your pelvis is naturally more tilted, you will need more tailbone energy; if you tend to be a tucker, you will need more pubic bone/groin deepening action. Almost nobody is naturally fifty-fifty, perfectly balanced, from the start. Throughout your practice your pelvis will change, so just like everything else in our practice, you have to keep checking in with this masculine/feminine conversation every day.

SHOULDERS AND ARMS

The shoulder and arm department is our main vehicle for nonverbal connection—waving, hugging, giving, and receiving. Since communication is best when it is a two-way street, let's explore how internal and external rotation in this area provides us with both outgoing and incoming possibilities.

Begin by letting your shoulders droop in toward your chest and let your upper body schlump. This posture is a big yoga don't. It's good to feel it now so you can recognize it if you ever drip down into that place again. The side effects of this position are shallow breathing and depression.

Here is how to correct this postural tendency. Stick your thumbs in your armpits as if you're at a hoedown pulling up your suspenders. Lift your armpits up and feel how that opens your chest. Keep your thumbs there and bring your middle fingers together at the center of your collarbones. Draw a line from there out to your shoulders, letting your collarbones broaden with the movement of your fingers.

Now slide your fingers and hands up and over your collarbones, just like a pizzamaker rolling a long roll of pizza dough. Let that pizza dough energy travel up and over the top of your shoulders. Let it flow down your back, tucking your shoulder blades into your rib cage.

Imagine your shoulder blades are two big warm hands on your back giving support to your heart and lungs (masculine). At the same time let your chest soften without sinking so that your back can be like the ground where your front rests (feminine).

Rub your hands together rapidly to create a little heat between your palms. Then place those warm hands on your kidneys, the area of your back between your ribs and pelvis, and let that heat from your hands melt and soften this area. Deepen your breath into your hands and feel how there is a possibility for width and expansion there. Begin to move your hands out to your sides and then wrap that energy around you like a snug cape that closes in the front, drawing the front ribs toward each other.

The lifting of the armpits and collarbones is external rotation, an opening action. The counteraction, wrapping the kidney cape, creates an internal direction that contains the outgoing energy. Explore how much you need of each to find harmony.

Stand in tadasana with your arms by your sides. Activate external rotation to bring your upper arm bones right into the middle of your shoulder sockets. With external rotation your palms will be facing away from your body. From your elbows to your fingertips, rotate your arms so your palms face the sides of your body. Be sure to maintain the external rotation of the upper arm to support the heart and lungs. This countertwist action balances the masculine and feminine in your arms. This holistic quality creates the ability to hold heavy things, including your own body, in weight-bearing activities.

The coordination of the masculine and feminine rotations in our upper body integrates our arms, shoulders, back, and rib cage. In turn, this alignment lets our arms support the heavenly organs of the heart and lungs and lets the back support the arms so they can become even more free, receptive, and expressive.

Our legs, pelvis, and hips are our main vehicle for locomotion or moving through our world. Our arms, shoulders, and chest are the primary method for communicating straight from the heart. When these two areas are balanced and in balance with each other, we can begin to join heaven and earth—our heart's aspirations with our grounded and directed action.

REMEMBER, NOT TOO TIGHT, NOT TOO LOOSE

When I was growing up I went to church every Sunday with my parents. There was a wonderful old lady there who was a big love bug. She always hugged everybody, especially me. In the early years I was captured and embraced by her belly and then eventually I moved up to being devoured by her generous bosom. In my teenage years I overheard her tell my mother that I used to put my head on her shelf but soon she would be putting her head on my shelf! I loved her but I have to admit that when she hugged me it was completely suffocating. Too tight for too long. These days I prefer an affectionate hug that brings two hearts together but still lets the lungs keep working.

Handshakes are almost the same as hugs—they're handhugs, and the same kind of syndrome arises. The limp dishrag handshake, where your hand almost falls out of the other person's: too loose. Or the macho handshake, where your fingers turn white: too tight. A good firm handshake allows for a two-way exchange and can be a very satisfying experience.

Just as we don't work too tightly or too loosely with our mind, we need to ride the middle path of effort and release in our muscular work as well.

Commonly asked questions in yoga class are: In this pose should I squeeze or release my buttocks? In this pose should I tighten or soften my abdominals? The answer is always the same—an enigmatic yes. Do both at the same time with the awareness that the degree of activation and release is different in various poses and with various people on various days.

What we are looking for is a way to be engaged without gripping. (Remember steadiness and ease?) I started thinking about this the night my boyfriend proposed to me. I felt happy that we were deepening our relationship but I didn't really relate to the concept of being engaged. I just thought you date, you live together, and then maybe you get married. Why bother being engaged for so long? But when Dave proposed to me, he said, "I want to be engaged with you. I want our lives together to be fully engaged, awake, and enlivened. There's no need to rush right to the next thing. Let's relish this in-between time to deeply engage in the richness of our lives together." I said, "Wow! OK."

Let's explore the experience of engaging our muscles as a continuous pulsation of active energy rather than a grasping that never changes (just the kind of marriage you wouldn't want!).

Stand in tadasana. Squeeze everything—your toes, your fingers, your face, your buttocks, your abdominals, all your muscles. Then let go and keep letting go until you schlump.

Now slowly, beginning from your feet, begin to rebuild tadasana, finding the middle path between clinging and detaching.

Press your feet and leg bones down into the earth as you affectionately hug your leg muscles onto your bones. Can you feel your leg muscles supporting the bones? Imagine that those same muscles are continuously flowing up, like socks being pulled on, as the bones burrow down.

Can you feel the pubic bone and tailbone relating to each other without hardening your groins, lower belly, or buttocks? How can you consciously energize these areas and still be open to the natural oscillations happening there today? It's okay if it's just in your mind and you're not sure you can feel anything. All this work begins with intention.

Now deepen your breathing and feel the movement of your chest, side ribs, and back. Can you explore this full breathing without letting your chest look like you just enlisted in the military?

Activate your arms. Hug the muscles up and onto the bones as you extend the bones out through the fingertips. Make karate chop hands. Make limp pasta hands. Now try to find middle path hands by letting each finger be a Buddha—awake.

Bobble your head around and try to find a point of balance where your head can sit on your neck. Let the skin all around the ring of your neck be even like a skin necklace made of pearls with an equal space between each bead.

Let your head be over your heart, your heart over your hips, your hips over your feet.

BUDDHA MIND

SUKHASANA

Asana practice means to place your body in a specific configuration and then sit with what arises. Every asana is the same in this respect. We can use the methods of joining heaven and earth, masculine and feminine coordination, and not too tight, not too loose in every pose. Each one of these contains an equal amount of physical awakening and mental attention. Form and content go hand in hand.

So the challenge of sukhasana (easy pose) is not just tying ourselves up like pretzels and plopping down on the floor. It includes our state of mind as we approach our practice, what arises when we are there, and how we relate to that. Let your meditation practice begin to infuse your asana practice by applying the meditation techniques of meeting your mind, watching the arc of your thoughts, and letting go of any project mentality or goal achievement. And then sometimes just let go of all of these instructions and don't worry. Exhale. Take a fresh start.

If yoga is called a practice, then what are we practicing and what are we practicing for? *Sukha* is sometimes translated as space. The opposite is *dukha*, which is sometimes translated as suffering, or by Krishnamacharya as "a dark room." In *The Solace of Open Spaces,* Gretel Ehrlich writes, "Space represents sanity, not a life purified, dull or 'spaced out' but one that might accommodate intelligently any idea or situation." Isn't that where we want to live?

FIVE

PATH WITHOUT A GOAL

Vinyasa Flow

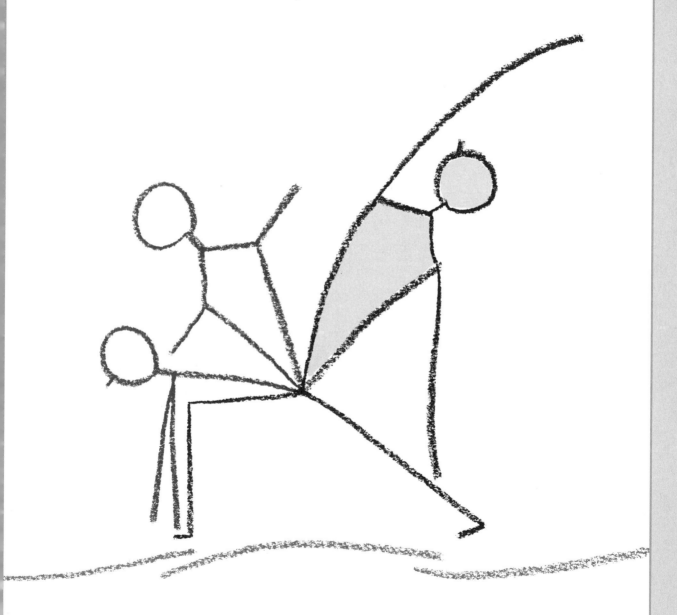

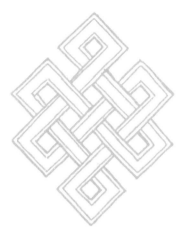

BUDDHA MIND

"You must destroy to create."
–Pablo Picasso

It's Friday night and I'm coasting the car down the ramp of Exit 70, but in my mind I'm already at the beach. I luxuriate in the texture of the sand as my toes celebrate freedom from winter's prison of shoes. I think about all the beach beings I've met—jellyfish, joggers, park rangers, cartwheeling kids, dogs and their identical people-parents—and the many sandy adventures my husband and I have had, including the usual headstand or two to look at the waves upside down. No matter what the weather, we rest our eyes on the horizon and our breath on the tide.

In reality, though, I'm still at the end of Exit 70, just coming up on the Mc-Donald's there. The vibrancy of my actual experiences at the beach are in my head, and in direct contrast to the hour-and-a-half drive it takes to get me there on the very long Long Island Expressway. I try to escape the boredom of the journey by listening to the radio, mentally processing my week, and engaging in other out-of-body activities that remove my mind from its premises.

But I question the wisdom of ignoring the huge portion of my life that is not a peak experience—not to mention the advisability of paying so little attention to my driving. How can I wake up to my own life at the same time that I am living it? And why would I want to?

When we get caught up in our thoughts we miss out on our life. It's as simple as that. In clichéd lingo we could say, "Stop and smell the roses." Just as I was planning my day at the beach before I even got off the freeway, we all have a tendency to mind-travel when we are bored by our ordinary activities. A very practical reason for being awake and present in our world is so we don't miss our exit on the freeway, or the moment when the next clothes dryer is available at the Laundromat or that handsome man steps into our life. It is true that for some of these mundane things we have cues, such as the oven timer, or the bank teller's voice saying, "Next!" But when we don't, we space out and miss out. This is like dropping out of your own life and when that happens, you become isolated from others.

Staying awake and present in our world, rather than creating our own thought-bubble existence, allows us to fully participate in the flow of traffic, the river of life, the ever-changing shape of our life. When we pay attention to our world, no matter how quickly it is changing (speeding down the freeway) or how slowly it is evolving (wrinkles and gray hair), we reaffirm our connection to all of life. This connection can be felt as a fullness that is also called yoga, which means union with everything, including *re*uniting with ourselves.

We all know this intuitively but remembering it is a challenge. That's why we practice repetitive activities such as watching our breath going in and out, over and over. Or walking in a circle. Or doing the sun salutation every single day. When we can begin to develop the concentration that is required to stay with these ordinary events, we will begin to notice the minute changes and inherent richness of our daily lives.

WALKING MEDITATION

Walking meditation is a technique for staying awake while moving through space. It's a way for us to realize that when we are moving we are still present, not just on the way to or from somewhere else. This is particularly helpful for people like me who do a lot of traveling on airplanes. Being up in the sky is literally ungrounding. It feels like you are nowhere, in a time and space limbo. The most popular solution is to do any old thing just to pass the time (and space)—watch the movie, read, fall asleep, eat more honey peanuts. Recently I have begun to look out the window at the vastness of the sky. It softens my brain fist and I am filled with the beauty of the phenomenal world—brilliant white cottony clouds and hot pink sun streaks. Instead of being dulled out by the canned air of the airplane, I begin to feel vibrant and alive by paying attention to every mountain peak, canyon river, and patchwork farm as I move through space.

The technique for walking meditation is almost the same as sitting meditation, but instead of using the breath as a landmark for staying present, we use the physical sensation of the feet on the floor as we walk, step by step. With your eyes open, gazing forward, you can begin to have a sense of the environment as you move through the world. Go slower than a normal walk, but not so slow that it is a labored, self-conscious activity. In fact, you can even do this walking down the street. You may see things on your block that you've never noticed in all the twenty years you've lived there.

Walking meditation helps us become aware of where we are right now, and how that changes with every breath, every step. It is traditionally done as part of longer meditation sessions as a relief for the body. After sitting for fifty or sixty minutes, meditators will walk for fifteen or twenty minutes. They usually walk in a circle or around the edges of the meditation hall. This also reminds us that we are not walking to get somewhere else. We are not meditating to get somewhere, either.

The practice of meditation is not a way to improve, be better, or get rid of anything, but to find out what's going on and fully experience that as it happens. As you continue to walk, the activity itself becomes its own raison d'être. Over time, this practice gradually cultivates curiosity and erodes task-oriented mentality. As you go around in a circle, you will begin to recognize landmarks— the shadow from the window, the texture of the loose floorboard, the sound of the radiator by the door—and to notice that, circle after circle, they stay the same and yet, they are different each time. And so are you.

Walking meditation is considered a transition practice between sitting meditation and infusing our daily activities with a sense of mindfulness. Sitting meditation is a formal practice that is important for stabilizing the mind and cultivating discipline. The time when we are not doing formal practice is called postmeditation and refers to all the rest of the twenty-four hours when we are not on our cushions. During those times, which is most of our life, it is recommended we cultivate a sense of meditative awareness. Walking meditation is a good step in that direction.

YOGA BODY

VINYASA ARISING, ABIDING, DISSOLVING

The day after I split from my first husband I met my second husband. I certainly did not know that was happening at that time. I only knew that the end of a phase had occurred. I felt sad but I also experienced a surge of fresh energy. I could feel that although one thing was ending, my whole life was not ending. Although I was certainly not on the lookout for a new boyfriend already, I did have a positive feeling that the ending I was experiencing was also the beginning of a new life for me. The great Zen master Eido Roshi once said, "Not knowing is the most intimate," and that was exactly how I felt—my senses were heightened and I felt very alive. In that open heart/mind state, I went to a party and met this really nice guy who asked me on a date the very next day. Eight years later, we were married.

When we practice asanas, we fold over, twist, turn upside down and inside out, place our body in specific shapes and stay there. During this process of repatterning our nervous system and reopening our pranic thoroughfares, we look to our breath and our mind for feedback on how we are doing on the tightrope of not too tight and not too loose. Throughout all this movement, we never leave our mat. We never go anywhere, except toward a recognition of who we are, starting with a deeper understanding of how we relate to our own body.

In the flowing form of vinyasa, each asana morphs into the next through choreographed movements that are based on the sun salutation sequence. Each body shape, each neurological circuit, each pulsation of effort and release flows into the next. We use the tidal quality of the breath to initiate each yoga movement and then join them all together in graceful sequences that place equal emphasis on the stillness of the asanas as well as the movement of the transitions.

In this way, vinyasa yoga becomes a physical practice that mirrors the cycling of all of life. Just like walking meditation is a way to begin to experience wakefulness as we move through our day, vinyasa yoga also cultivates awareness of our environment as well as the curiosity and confidence to be open to whatever might arise in the next moment.

To the uninitiated observer, it may appear as though the yogi is completely stationary as he or she "holds" a pose. In actuality, yoga asanas are not static events at all. Each yoga pose has three parts: 1) moving into the pose; 2) abiding in the pose; and 3) coming out of the pose. Yoga philosophy calls this creation, maintenance, and destruction.

The longer flow of a vinyasa sequence is an extension of the three parts of every pose—arising, abiding, and dissolving. In this case, at the same time that you are moving out of one pose—dissolving—you are simultaneously moving into the next—arising. In other words, part 3 of the first pose is the same as part 1 of the next pose. This fluid approach to yoga asana practice is how we start to understand that the "in-between" moments of building and letting go that are part 1 and part 3 are just as important as the experience of abiding in part 2. Especially since there are more parts 1 and 3 than parts 2 anyway.

When we practice paying attention to every breath, to every step, to every pose and the transitions in between, we begin to understand that in fact, everything is in between and each moment is of equal value. There is no peak experience and no nonpeak experience. Driving on the expressway might not be a peak experience, but if I wake up to the vividness of the cars, the city mutating into the country, the energy of fast motion, it reminds me that every moment of our lives is valuable.

When we apply our mindfulness to our vinyasa practice, we begin to really see what is in front of us and to watch how it transforms with every breath. As one thing flows into the next, we begin to understand experientially the vastness of our connectivity and the power of every moment. This awareness cuts through our attachment to project mentality because it's not task-oriented. In vinyasa yoga, you're never finished because every ending is a beginning. It is a physical expression of path without a goal.

SURYA NAMASKAR (SUN SALUTE)

Beginning with this chapter I offer you several yoga sequences you can do every day or as often as you like. The repetitive aspect of the practice is boring and fascinating at the same time. Imagine if you paid really close attention while brushing your teeth every morning. You would start to notice tiny shifts in the color and texture of the enamel, the tenderness of the gums, and subtle changes in all the little bumps and smooth parts of your teeth. You would get incredibly familiar with your own mouth. But we don't do that. We just get through it, all the while planning what else we have to do that day.

Doing the same old sun salutation day in and day out provides us the opportunity to change that pattern. Waking up to every single breath, every single moment, is the challenge of this flowing form of yoga. To include every sensation whether it comes under the category of pleasant or not. To let go of categories. To let go of the fruits of your action. To literally go with the flow. This is the path to equanimity.

The following sequences are variations of the sun salute, the primary vinyasa sequence of yoga asana practice. In many traditions it is the standard way to begin daily yoga class. In OM yoga, which is a vinyasa or flowing style of yoga, the sun salute sequence is used to connect many of the poses throughout the entire class so that the yogini experiences how everything is connected all the time—breath, movement, body, mind, up, down, in, and out.

There are many benefits to the sun salute. It is a series of alternating backward and forward bends, creating a balance of energy and awareness in the relationship between the front and back of our body. As this relationship deepens, the sun salute becomes a practice of finding the support and courage to open the heart (backbending), and then softening back into our core and resting the brain (forward bending).

The sun salute is a way for us to remember and give thanks for the life-giving qualities of the sun. It organically reminds us of our connection to the sun because intense heat is generated through the continuous movement. You will get hot and sweaty, which feels quite purifying, like taking a bath from the inside out. It is also important to remember that sunlight is part of the rhythm of night and day. Although the sun salute is an active sequence, try to incorporate the receptive aspect of the full cycle of life, extending out energetically, yet being receptive to the world you are moving through.

How do you do this? By combining equal amounts of bright observation with a quality of relaxation that allows you to open to your own sensuous experience. Observing is opening out to your environment, hearing your breath, feeling the mat beneath you and the sweat on your skin, watching your thoughts and seeing what is in front of you no matter which way your head is pointing. Relaxing is riding the wave of the movement and not worrying. It's only yoga, remember? In addition to cultivating strength in the entire body, and enhancing heart and lung activity, the sun salute is fun!

BUDDHA MIND

TRAVELING TADASANA: A MOVING MEDITATION

The alignment instructions for the individual asanas within the sun salute sequence never vary from the basic information you learned about tadasana. In fact, you could say that the vinyasa is all one tadasana, which transforms over and over in endless variations.

As you move through this traveling tadasana, find the connection of heaven and earth by reaching your leg bones down into the earth as you draw the muscles and skin of your legs up, like pulling long stockings all the way up to your hips. Feel an oppositional relationship between your tailbone and the crown of your head. Balance your head over your heart and your heart over your hips.

Continue to explore the conversation between your pubic bone and tailbone. This is an ongoing oscillation that gets more refined over time until eventually you may experience both the tilt and the tuck of the pelvis at the same time, leading to an energetic lift of the front of the spine. For now, let the deepening of the groins and the dropping of the tailbone be a dialogue between front and back, a balancing of feminine and masculine energies.

Remind yourself about the fluid relationship between the external rotation that opens the chest, lifts the collarbones, and supports the heart and lungs, with the internal rotation that broadens the back waist and fills the kidney area with breath and energy.

Each movement, asana, and transition should take as long as each breath, so you never stop breathing or moving. Try to make your inhalations and exhalations slow and equal in length, so that your movements are balanced. Moving with the breath requires that all parts of the body work in harmony, teaching us rhythm, coordination, and gracefulness. The idea is to use your breath as a home base, just as in meditation technique, to experience the richness of each moment, whether it's challenging, strenuous, energizing, or relaxing. Let your body unfold on each breath.

If you want to stay in any position for more than one breath, that's fine. When you are "holding" a pose, that doesn't mean there is no movement. Each asana itself is a mini vinyasa. This is a good time to review and refine the tadasana information: extending out in all directions and falling back to center; balancing inner awareness and outer vision; reaching up and down; equalizing the breath in your front, back, and sides; activating your muscles; and softening your sense organs. When you do all this with mindfulness, it is not exercise, but a moving meditation.

Let your vinyasa practice remind you of the preciousness of every moment of every day. Then after your yoga class, try to carry a sense of postmeditative awareness out into the rest of your day. You can start by doing walking meditation on the street after your yoga class so that your vinyasa practice becomes the model for experiencing the fullness of life all the time.

YOGA BODY

SUN SALUTE SEQUENCES (SURYA NAMASKAR)

We begin every class at OM Yoga Center with a warm-up vinyasa and then move into sun salutes. I have included a warm-up vinyasa sequence here, which you can use as your sun salute if you are a brand-new beginner.

BRAND-NEW BEGINNER SUN SALUTE, OR WARM-UP VINYASA

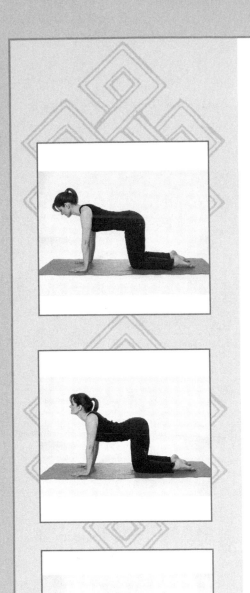

1. Hands and Knees

Make sure that your wrists are directly below your shoulders and your knees are directly below your hips. Take a glance at the crease of your wrist and make sure it is parallel to the edge of your mat. Using this guideline, point either your index finger or your middle finger straight ahead and fan your fingers out from there like wide-5s. Don't go so wide that your baby fingers turn white!

2. *Bitilasana* • Cow

As you inhale, drop your belly, letting your spine absorb into your body and creating an arch in your back. Reach your sitting bones up as you open your chest. Keep your collarbones wide apart and some length in the back of your neck. Try not to scrunch your forehead here.

3. *Bitilasana* • Cat

As you exhale, reverse this spinal curve, lifting your navel up toward your spine. Tuck your pelvis under and drop your head. Still try to keep some space in the throat and broadness in the collarbones.

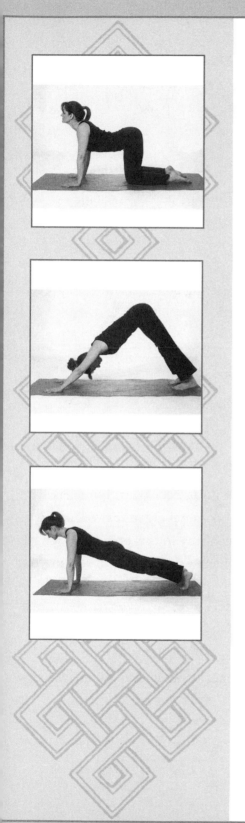

4. *Bitilasana* • Cow

Inhale, as you once again tilt your pelvis upward and lengthen the front of the vertebrae.

5. *Adho Mukha Svanasana* • Downward-Facing Dog

Keep the cow tilt in your pelvis as you move into downward-facing dog. Press your hands down to make the opposing action of the hips lifting. Extend down through your heels—they do not have to touch the floor—as you reach up through your sitting bones.

6. Plank

Keep reaching out through your heels as you begin to take your shoulders forward coming into plank pose. Let your abdominal wall fly up so that it supports your spine without getting too hard. Activate your leg and arm muscles strongly.

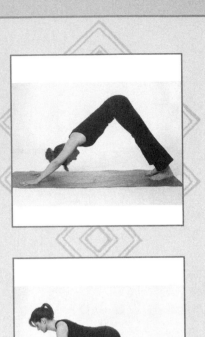

7. *Adho Mukha Svanasana* • Downward-Facing Dog

Let your thigh bones draw you back into downward-facing dog. Try not to let your armpits droop like a hammock.

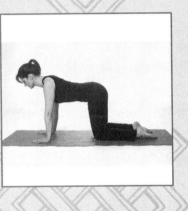

8. Hands and Knees

Keep reaching up with your sitting bones as you gently lower your knees back to the floor.

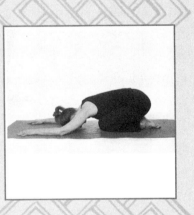

9. *Balasana* • Child's Pose

Point your feet and press your hips back over your heels. This is a nice massage for your abdominal organs as well as a resting pose for the brain. You can stay in this pose for as long as you want. Use this pose whenever you need to rest in your practice.

From child's pose you can come right back onto hands and knees again, making this sequence a continuous loop. Eventually try to do this sequence at least four times in a row - straight through.

BEGINNER SUN SALUTE

Practice letting the end of one asana be the beginning of the next. Take your time and feel everything along the way.

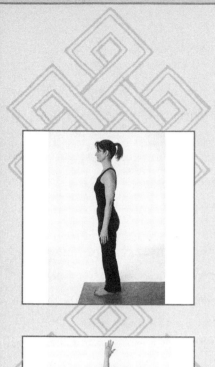

1. *Tadasana* • Mountain Pose

Stand firmly on the four corners of your feet. Drop your weight down into the floor and feel your spine lifting up in response, all the way up through the top of your head. Soften your eyes, ears, the root of your tongue.

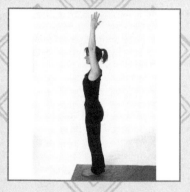

2. *Urdhva Hastasana* • Arms Up

inhale

Extend through the fingers as you circle your arms out to the sides and all the way up next to your ears. Look for a lift in the back ribs while letting the front ribs stay soft. As the chest opens upward let your gaze fly up to the space between your hands.

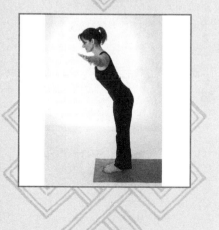

3. Swan Dive

exhale

Reverse the circle of the arms. Check that you don't let your arms fly back behind you but instead make sure that you maintain the connection of the shoulder blades on the back, allowing the arms to go directly out from the sideline of your shoulders.

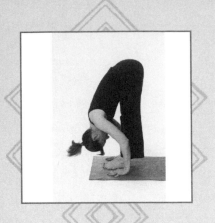

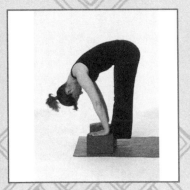

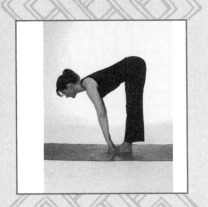

4. *Uttanasana 1* • Standing Forward Bend

exhale

This is the ending moment of the swan dive. As you fold over your legs, find the balance between a lengthening feeling in the legs and activating the muscles of the legs, drawing them up the bones. If you can't feel that, run your hands up your leg muscles, encouraging that lifted sensation. Relax the back of your neck and let your head drop.

Variation with blocks: If you feel tight anywhere along the back of your body, including the soles of the feet, backs of the leg, back of the torso, neck, and the scalp all the way up around and over to the place between your eyebrows—then bend your knees or place your hands on blocks. The bend should happen right at the top of your legs, not at your waist.

5. *Uttanasana 2* • Standing Forward Bend with Flat Back

inhale

Extend the sitting bones back and lengthen the spine. This first time you try this you can touch your sternum with one hand and your tailbone with the other and imagine them lengthening away from each other. If you feel tight anywhere on the back of your body, which includes your neck, back, hamstrings, and the soles of your feet, then bend your knees as much as you need to in order to release that tension and open the chest.

Don't forget about your hands. Every finger should be awake, whether you are touching the floor with flat hands, fingertips, the front of your shins, or yoga blocks.

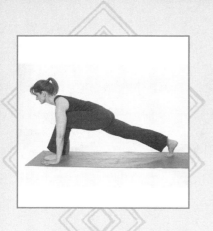

6. Lunge

exhale

Step back with your right leg. Find the strength of the back leg and lift the thigh toward the ceiling at the same time that you soften in the front of the left hip. It's a lot to think about so take your time and keep breathing.

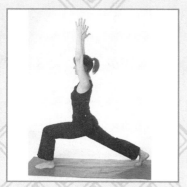

7. *Virabhadrasana 1 Preparation* • High Lunge

inhale

Before you lift your spine, take a moment here to touch your tailbone. Then replace your hand to the floor. Feel your two thighs moving away from each other and drop your tailbone into the space that creates. Let that downward action of the tailbone begin the movement of lifting your spine up into the high lunge.

Variation: Keep lifting up through the crown of your head and every single finger as you bend your back knee slightly. With the back knee bent, lift your hip points, bringing your pelvis into a more vertical alignment. Try to maintain that placement as you extend out through the back heel to straighten the leg again. Watch what happens to your rib cage. Your front ribs may have a tendency to flare open so use your abdominals to draw them inward and think of lengthening in your back waist. Repeat this exercise a few times, exploring the opening in the front hip area of the back leg. This exercise will help you learn how to balance the pelvis and organize the relationship between your hips and ribs. It will also create tremendous strength in your legs.

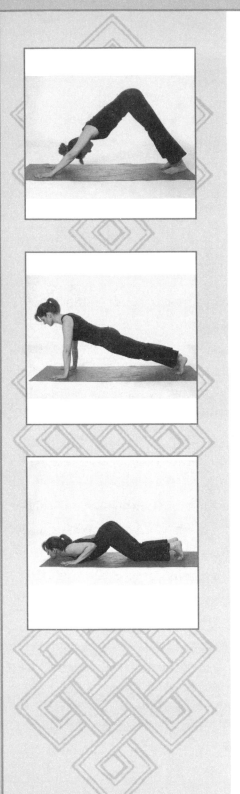

8. *Adho Mukha Svanasana* • Downward-Facing Dog

exhale

Place your palms on the floor and lift your hips into downward-facing dog pose. Reach your arms into the floor like Superman and lift your hips up as high as you can.

9. Plank

inhale

Reach the crown of your head forward as you lengthen your tailbone back.

10. *Astang Pranam* • Knees-Chest-Chin

exhale

This is like a worm doing a backbend. Keep your sitting bones lifting high as you lower your chest and chin to the floor. There is a tendency when learning this transition to lower your chest straight down to the floor. Be brave and move it forward into the space right between your hands. If your arms are not strong yet, you might plop down a little bit at first, but that's okay. Make sure your elbows are pointing straight back, not out to the sides like in a pushup. Press all ten fingers down and lift your shoulders up away from your index knuckles.

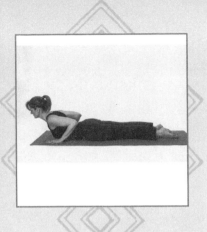

11. *Bhujangasana* • Baby Cobra

inhale

Drop the pelvis and let that initiate the movement to slide forward into this upper chest opener. Let the bottom ribs stay on the floor. Try not to grip your buttocks, but do activate the legs and reach out through all ten toes. Keep your collarbones broad and maintain some length in the back of the neck.

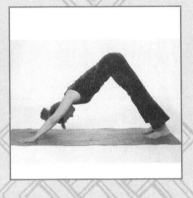

12. *Adho Mukha Svanasana* • Downward-Facing Dog

exhale

Use your legs to take some of the weight off the arms. If your low back or legs feel tight, bend your knees slightly but keep extending your sitting bones up to the sky so your pelvis becomes a giant blossoming flower. Let your belly be soft and feel your breath moving there. Stay here for three to eight breaths.

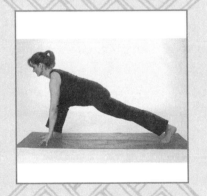

13. Step Forward into a Lunge

exhale

Make this movement on an exhale so your belly softens and there is room for your thigh. If your foot doesn't get all the way into the space between your hands, no problem. Take hold of it with your hand and shift it forward. Over time your hips will open and you'll easily step right into place.

14. Gap

inhale

Stay here and rest your mind for one breath.

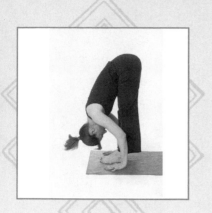

15. *Step Forward into Uttanasana 1* • Standing Forward Bend

exhale

Step your back foot forward to meet the other foot and fold right over into a standing forward bend. Again, bend your knees if the back of your body is tight.

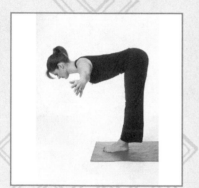

16. Reverse Swan Dive

inhale

Press your feet down and let that begin to lift you all the way back up.

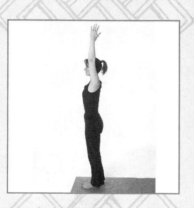

17. *Urdhva Hastasana* • Arms Up

Look at the space between your hands and then notice if your fingers are alive. Can you keep your throat soft here?

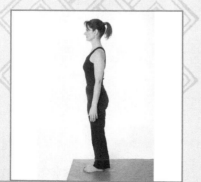

18. *Tadasana* • Mountain Pose

exhale

Back to home base. How is it different from the first tadasana of this sequence?

Repeat entire sequence with the left leg.

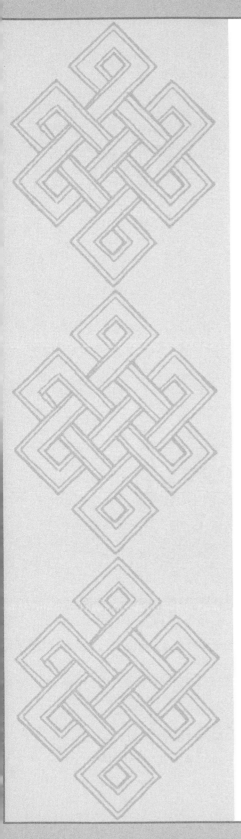

INTERMEDIATE SUN SALUTE

At this level you begin to learn jumpings and develop the strength for chaturanga.

1. *Tadasana* • Mountain Pose

Find the balance of front and back, up and down. (Pictured on page 67.)

2. *Urdhva Hastasana* • Arms Up

inhale

Initiate the lift of the arms from the bottom of the shoulder blades, as if your arms were wings coming right out of your heart. (Pictured on page 67.)

3. *Swan Dive into Uttanasana 1* • (Standing Forward Bend)

exhale

Lift your sitting bones up as the crown of head reaches down. Make sure to fold right at the top of your legs where your bikini line is. If it feels like your belt is on too tight when you bend, it means you need to bend your legs. (Pictured on page 67–68.)

4. *Uttanasana 2* • Forward Bend with Long Spine

inhale

Let the breath fill your back and sides as well as the front of your body. (Pictured on page 77.)

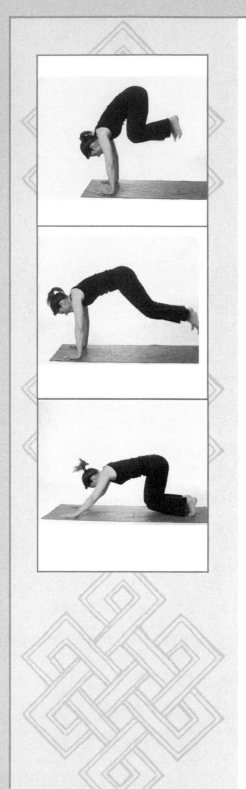

5. Jump Back

exhale

Bend your knees a lot, jump up, and make sure to bend your knees a lot when you land.

6. *Adho Mukha Svanasana* • Downward-Facing Dog

same exhale

Look for equal weight on arms and legs. (Pictured on page 65.)

7. Plank

inhale

Take your gaze slightly forward to allow your neck to continue the two-way extension of the spine. (Pictured on page 65.)

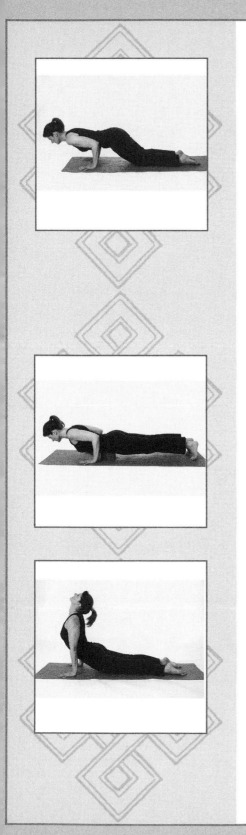

8. Upper Body Chaturanga

exhale

Come onto all fours with a neutral spine, neither curved nor arched. Keep the sitting bones reaching back as you begin to bend your elbows straight back, taking your chest slightly forward in space. Do not let your shoulders get lower than your elbows.

From here, you can straighten your arms and repeat this chaturanga variation several times to develop upper body strength. Or you can do it once and collapse in a heap. Rest, and then move on to upward-facing dog pose. Or you can work on the following exercise to practice chaturanga.

Learning how to do chaturanga: Place a block under your pelvis. Align your wrists under your elbows. Strengthen and lengthen your legs so much that the thighs lift off the floor. Reach your tailbone down toward your pubic bone so your buttocks is not sticking up. Roll your shoulders back, lift your head, and look slightly forward. On an inhale, inflate your back waist and lift off the block. Stay here and try to breathe for three breaths. Whew!

9. *Urdhva Mukha Svanasana* • Upward-Facing Dog

inhale

Dive forward with the same kind of action as moving into baby cobra from astang pranam (knees-chest-chin). Lift your thighs up. Nothing is touching the floor here except the palms of your hands and the tops of your feet.

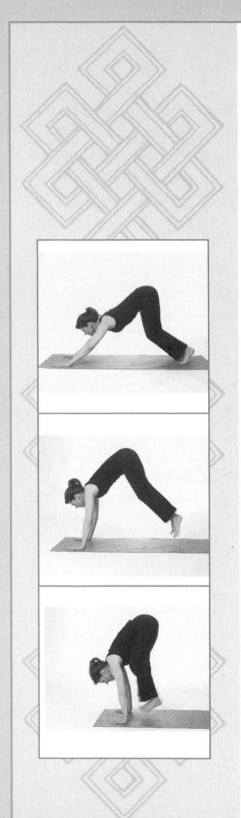

10. *Adho Mukha Svanasana* • Downward-Facing Dog

exhale

Float your pelvis up and let that lightness help you roll right over the tops of your feet into downward-facing dog. It's important to go over your two feet together, not one at a time, so your pelvis doesn't get habitually twisted. Stay here for three to five breaths. (Pictured on page 65.)

11. Jump Forward

exhale

Near the end of your last exhale in downward-facing dog, bend your knees and look at the space between your hands. That is where your feet are going to land. Go! Don't worry if you don't get all the way there. Take two jumps if you need to, and just keep practicing.

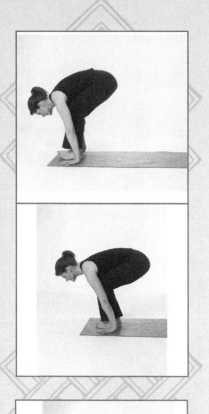

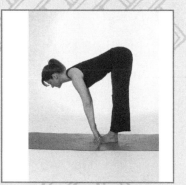

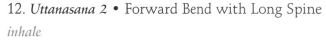

12. *Uttanasana 2* • Forward Bend with Long Spine

inhale

Land from the jump with bent knees and then let the inhalation lift you up into this-flat back position.

13. *Uttanasana 1* • Standing Forward Bend

exhale

Keep your legs strong and your arms and hands active as you release your spine and neck.

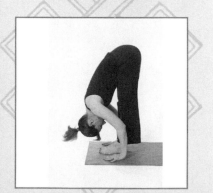

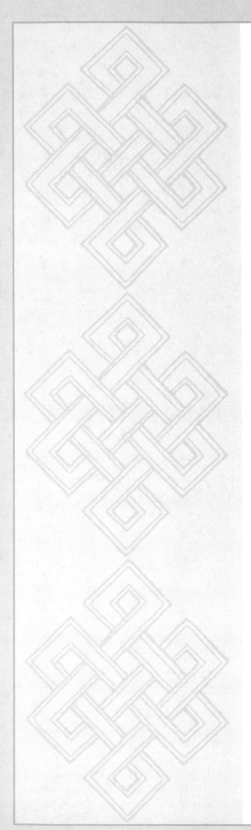

14. *Reverse Swan Dive into Urdhva Hastasana* • (Arms Up)
inhale
Let the feet and hands be bright. (Pictured on page 72.)

15. *Tadasana* • Mountain Pose
exhale
Feel the top of your head lifting up as your arms float down by your sides. (Pictured on page 72.)

ADVANCED SUN SALUTE
This sun salute is the most rigorous variation.

1. *Tadasana* • Mountain Pose
inhale and exhale
Let this pose remind you to come to attention while opening your sensory organs. (Pictured on page 67.)

2. *Urdhva Hastasana* • Arms Up
inhale
Lift the back ribs to begin floating the arms upward. (Pictured on page 67.)

3. *Swan Dive into Uttanasana 1 (Standing Forward Bend)*
exhale
Dive through the ocean of air all around you. Try not to let your sitting bones shift back behind you as you fold in half. (Pictured on page 67 and 68.)

4. *Uttanasana 2* • Forward Bend with Long Spine
inhale

Move the spaces in your groins away from the spaces in your armpits. (Pictured on page 68.)

5. *Jump Back into Chaturanga Dandasana (Four-Limbed Stick Pose)*
exhale

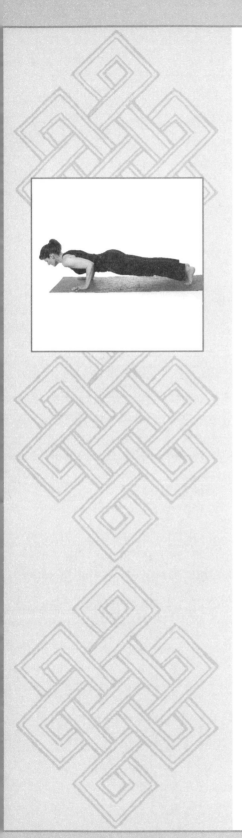

Keep your spine reaching forward as your legs shoot back, landing right in chaturanga.

Firm the shoulder blades on the back to protect your shoulders as you transition into the next pose.

6. *Urdhva Mukha Svanasana* • Upward-Facing Dog
inhale

Can you have a sense of breath broadening the back of the waist and pelvis? (Pictured on page 75.)

7. *Adho Mukha Svanasana* • Downward-Facing Dog
three to five breaths

Put helium balloons in your hips and loft them high to roll over the feet in this pose. (Pictured on page 65.)

Find your breath here. Try not to apply a special breathing technique, but allow your breath to be a mirror that reflects your own mental and energetic experience back to you.

8. Jump Forward
exhale

At the end of your last exhale, bend the knees and float the pelvis up and forward, landing lightly, like a butterfly on a

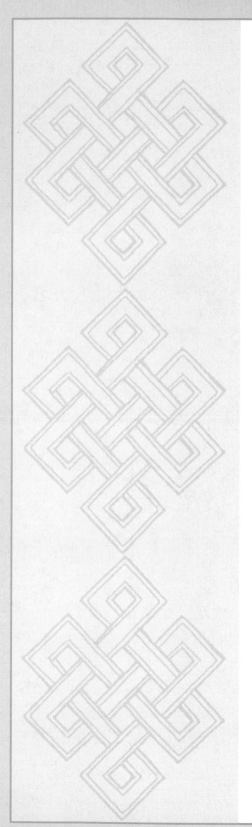

lily pad. That will take some practice. Try to get your shoulders over your wrists as soon as possible and that will help you to fly. (Pictured on page 76.)

9. *Uttanasana 2* • Forward Bend with Long Spine
inhale
Press the feet down to find the lift of the sitting bones. Lengthen the spine in two directions and softly fill the lungs. (Pictured on page 77.)

10. *Uttanasana 1* • Standing Forward Bend
exhale
Let the breath pour out of you like a waterfall as your spine cascades over your legs. (Pictured on page 77.)

11. Reverse Swan Dive into Urdhva Hastasana (Arms Up)
inhale
Feel your in-breath lift you like the wind lifts a kite. (Pictured on page 72.)

12. *Tadasana* • Mountain Pose
exhale
Find the balance between coming to attention and relaxing with what is. (Pictured on page 72.)

SIX

HOW TO BE A WARRIOR

Standing Poses

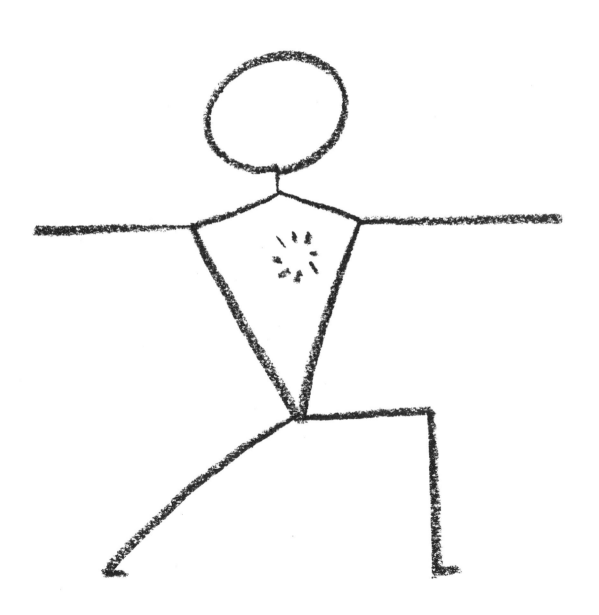

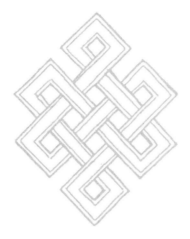

Yoga Body

What is strong and what is weak? Have you ever been crushed by a dirty look or melted by a smile? How is it that a blade of grass can crack the sidewalk to grow up to the sun? How is it that the falling snow can break a tree branch? How can we find the balance of both inner and outer strength? And how can we make our yoga practice both an athletic work-out and a meditative work-in?

Just as sitting meditation helps tame and stabilize our wild mind, asana practice often begins with standing poses, which strengthen and stabilize the legs and arms. These are considered the organs of action in yoga and when they are fully functional—strong and properly aligned—they provide the fluid, yet stable base necessary to support the heart, lungs, visceral organs, and vertebral column.

Standing poses are physically challenging and it doesn't take long before your legs begin to quiver, your body gets warm, and your arms feel very heavy. That is fine. That is the natural process that we human beings have to go through to develop muscular strength. The problem that sometimes arises is that when we work hard on a physical level, we tend to get hard in our minds and hearts, too.

Have you ever watched bodybuilding competitions on TV? Those guys and gals grunt freely and frequently. There is no question that a lot of effort is required to lift those big, round metal things up in the air. The cause and effect relationship is clear—you have to push, pull, and pump really hard to get a strong, fit body. There is no magic pill, no secret weapon. Only continuous sweat and strain. It's a one-dimensional highway to hunkville. This makes sense to many of us. We tend to think that exercise is supposed to be intense and so we work too hard. But then the activity itself becomes too hard and so do we.

Although it is obvious that mainstream America values big strong bodies, I was still surprised by a serious meditator friend who confessed that the reason he has resisted yoga is he doesn't have time to add another thing to his life. He chose to stick with the gym because he's afraid that by only doing that wimpy yoga stuff he will lose the hunky physique he has worked so hard to obtain. There are Chinese tai chi masters who would call this Westerner a lobster—hard on the outside, but no inner strength. These guys are called masters because they can knock you across the room with an exhale.

We know that yoga asanas are not easy; they take physical effort and concentration. So why isn't the yogini's face contorted like the weightlifter's? At first, sometimes it is. Even though I teach my yoga students to engage their organs of action, the arms and legs, I often see them trying to get through the standing poses by screwing up their mouths, gripping their butts, tensing their fingers and toes, and bugging out their eyes. All these responses are the same ones we make in our everyday lives when things come up that push our buttons, frighten or overwhelm us. We grip our mouths, butts, and toes. Then we either ignore the whole thing or we armor ourselves inwardly to be able to take on the challenge. Naturally, this is the same thing we do in yoga class. Fortunately, when we become aware of this ineffective tendency, our yoga practice can become an opportunity to reverse our habitual response to difficulty.

I have to admit that standing poses are not my favorite. It's easier for me to sit down, fold in half, and watch my breath. There's a reason why some of them are called warrior poses and not powderpuff poses. If you've ever tried them before, you probably know what I'm talking about. Standing poses are usually done near the beginning of a class and that's about when I start thinking that I should go to the bathroom, or that I need to make a phone call, or the more honest "I hate these poses." But I never do leave and later, of course, I'm always glad I did myself the favor of sticking with it.

Unlike weightlifting, yoga's standing poses will eventually stimulate your digestive system, strengthen your heart and lungs, and purify and nourish your spleen, intestines, liver, and kidneys. These benefits will happen to a certain degree even without us knowing it, which is good since most of us cannot feel this internal toning as easily as we can feel our muscle groups firing as they grow stonger. Unfortunately, you won't get as much benefit if your body gets too hard on the outside, because the overworked muscles harden your internal organs, which then get dry and tight and lose proper functionality.

Overly tight chest, shoulder, and back muscles restrict the range of motion in the upper body, which will diminish heart and lung activity. Abdominal hardness, pulling the navel back in toward the spine, squishes the digestive and reproductive organs, leading to both emotional and digestive constipation. A highly contracted core body loses its ability for healthy movement and ultimately shows up through mental obstacles, like feeling crabby, or physical tension that can turn into migraines.

Of course, it takes a certain level of mental and physical effort to practice standing poses. In the Yoga Sutra of Patanjali this kind of focused exertion is called tapas, and it is one of the important niyamas, or guiding principles, of yoga. *Tapas* is translated as "fire" or "heat" and refers to the sustained discipline and commitment needed to walk the path of the yogi. The idea of a burning fire or passion for the practice is inspiring for many of us, and it's what keeps us coming back to the mat. Tapas helps us ignite the hearth of yoga and connect to the brilliance and luminosity of this beautiful practice. But it is important to note that this fervor can also get out of balance and become a form of pride in accomplishment—"I haven't missed a day of practice in ten years!"—as well as a form of fever, which is the quickest way to burn out on yoga and give it up altogether.

The only way to keep the flame burning without getting too bright or too dim is to pay attention to the process and be honest with yourself. That is the practice. The real challenge of these poses is to discover the exact amount of tapas—focus, effort, and awareness—that allows us to abide in these positions without mentally or physically dropping out of the intensity of the experience altogether (burnout), or without putting our heart, mind, and body in a choke-hold and just hanging on until it's over (spiritual pride).

Donna Farhi, renowned yoga teacher and author of *Yoga Mind, Body and Spirit,* translates *tapas* as "burning enthusiasm." When I am tempted to drop out of standing poses either physically or mentally, I remind myself that I do have enthusiasm for the practice, that I do have faith in the benefits of yoga, that I can be a warrior as I do warrior poses. How do I cultivate the tapas of a warrior, not too hot and not too cold, that gives me the discipline to stay seated in the saddle of my pelvis and ride steady through the waves of craving, irritation, and exhilaration?

I let the challenge of the warrior poses remind me of the path of the sacred warrior, an ancient code of conduct that, according to Chögyam Trungpa Rinpoche, "is available to any human who seeks a genuine and fearless existence." The inspiration of the sacred warrior invites me to cut through my discursive thinking and have the courage to stay connected to my full range of feeling by using the warrior's weapons of precision, gentleness, opening, and natural intelligence.

Buddha Mind

Precision

After the first few breaths in a standing pose, you may begin to notice an initial sensory experience of burning quadriceps which then becomes a thought such as,

"This is not my favorite pose," which turns into an entire story line—"Why does this teacher always hold this pose so long? I don't think I'm going to take this teacher's class again because she talks too much during this pose and I really don't know if it's good to stay here this long, maybe I will just straighten this leg and pretend to check out my front knee alignment and stall for time, I really prefer seated poses and they are probably better for me personally anyway, since I've been working so hard lately and I think I'm going to have a glass of wine with dinner tonight because I really need to pamper myself because I just never get enough sleep and that's why this is so hard for me and I can't believe that this teacher is still having us hold this pose. . . ." Or the story line might be, "I am going to hold this pose no matter what. I'm going to ignore that sharp twinge in my back knee and even though my arms are starting to shake I'm staying here. Oh, remember to breathe. I don't think I can really breathe too deeply here, maybe I'll make my breathing get louder and harder, and squeeze my butt more. There's no way I'm going to be the first person to drop out of this pose!" Sound familiar?

One of the keys to unlocking our mental soap operas is precision. Precision is the warrior's sword that cuts through our dramas and resistance. Working with precision in our yoga and meditation practice is extemely helpful, because it creates form, and form creates space. Sometimes people have the opposite idea about precision—that it implies being shut down, boxed in. In one of my yoga classes I asked the students to do the sun salute with precision. Then to do it a second time with grace. I asked them which they preferred and gracefulness was the unanimous winner. They said the precise version felt harsh, militaristic, tight, rigid, icky, cold, boring, and dead. One person said she thought of precision and perfection as the same thing, and since that seems unavailable, she felt like precision was self-defeating.

"What if you make a clean slice in a bagel?" I asked. "Does that seem rigid and unfeeling or simply a useful method for preparing breakfast?" The group revelation was that their ideas about precision were what was bogging them down. That, in fact, their relationship to the notion of precision was actually . . . imprecise. As they realized that precision was neither good nor bad, but simply a helpful tool or strategy, they eagerly offered new synonyms for precision, moving through exact and clean and settling on clear as their favorite. The discovery of precision as clarity gave them a feeling of new beginning, of opening, of space.

Precision is a way to develop clarity of mind at the same time that we develop accuracy in our physical placement. Applying specificity to where you put your hands and feet creates a wakeful mental attitude. You simply can't think clearly if your alignment is sloppy. For example, what is your posture right now as you are reading this? Try changing your position, or even walking around and see if you feel sleepy or clear.

It is also difficult to feel openhearted or uplifted if your chest is sunk and your spine is sagging. Not only are your cardiovascular functions diminished, but your body is a cage. This curling in creates dukha, suffering, which is the opposite of sukha, space, and both can relate to the physical and emotional space created through good (or poor) posture. Hatha yoga aligns skin, muscles, and bones so that each can support the other with as much ease as effort. Proper alignment opens energetic blockages, which can be caused by diet, stress, illness, and emotions.

Physical precision extends to your clothing (think twice about tight belts, wristwatches, and excess fabric flapping around your head in yoga class), environment, personal hygiene, and how to arrange your practice space. Organize your mat and yoga props—blankets, blocks, straps—in a neat and orderly fashion because a jumbled heap of stuff in your line of sight creates an obstacle as well. Everybody who has a messy desk knows this to be true. The discipline of precision can help establish a sense of open heart, open mind, and open agenda. Form creates space.

As you work with standing poses, try to notice when your body gets tired or your mind gets bored. Stick with it anyway. When it feels difficult, don't try too hard but instead apply just the necessary amount and qualities of right action: rhythm, movement, direction, energy, and intention, but never aggression. This kind of precision is in line with the warrior's code of having the courage to face reality and relate to it appropriately.

GENTLENESS

Just as many of us cringe at the notion of precision, the word *warrior* can positively make us recoil in disgust. As yogis we may base our life on the very first ground principle of yoga, which is ahimsa—not harming self or others. How can a warrior have anything to do with ahimsa? In the Buddhist context, a warrior is not someone who conquers others. Rather a sacred warrior is one who cultivates fearlessness by looking straight at their own fears without judgment or aggression, with bravery and kindness to oneself. This kind of gentleness is the seed for growing a warrior's heart. It doesn't mean being a pushover. It means seeing with precision what is happening here and now in any given situation and then having the courage to open our beating heart to that. When we approach our yoga asanas with the precision and gentleness of the warrior, our practice becomes a training program for being centered, awake, confident, and flexible within challenging situations.

Recently I got a letter from a man in prison. This man's journey has led him to understand that his greatest strength was to be openhearted. He wrote:

Ms. Cyndi Lee,

For the last year and a half, I've been trying to point my life down a positive path. It's been an arduous adventure, uphill all the way. Still I struggle.

When I read through your piece on the Warrior Poses . . . I realized that part of my reluctance to leading a positive, pro-social life was a fear of being weak, or being seen that way by contemporaries.

In my childhood, all life was a struggle. I quickly developed into a dominant, aggressive, alpha-male type. It took a long time and a lot of hardship and self-destructive activity to figure out that doesn't work too well.

[Now] I realize that I can still be a strong warrior at heart, without letting that bleed off into my social life as aggression and anti-social stubbornness.

Being a strong warrior at heart doesn't mean being wimpy, although this is what this man feared other people's perceptions might be. In the case of the sacred warrior, gentleness means absence of doubt, which translates into confidence. This is different from arrogance, which is another form of fear, and often has a point to prove or a score to settle. Real confidence invites us to let go of doubt, even though we might feel our leg muscles burning and our arms quivering, or we might feel threatened, alone, or abandoned.

When we remember our relationship to earth and heaven—earth is always there and will let anyone sit on it and heaven is always above you as a reminder of the vastness of your own nature—then we can rest in a profound sense of confidence based on the simple fact that we are born and we are good. We don't have to prove ourselves, be tough, be hard or soft, or be any different from exactly who we are already right now. This relaxed confidence doesn't need to be aggressive, but can be brave enough to be gentle in all situations. Precision, which helps us cut through the thickness of neuroses, to open up space to see clearly, coupled with gentleness, which helps us relate to our situation without habitual aggression, grasping, or ignoring, will lead us toward experiencing the true power of the warrior.

OPENING

The third weapon of the warrior is the courage to stay open. Prominent yoga teacher Erich Schiffmann, author of *Yoga: The Spirit and Practice of Moving into Stillness,* says that to expand is not egotistical but to shrink is. We have already seen how precision opens up space and how gentleness opens up opportunities that would be shut down if we approached them with aggression. But how do we stay open? What does that mean—physically and mentally?

There is a popular notion of yoga as a stretching activity. Sure, there are muscle-lengthening movements in asana practice, but yoga is not really about stretching. One of my favorite yoga teachers, Judith Lasater, author of *Relax and Renew* and *Living Your Yoga,* said, "The only thing that can create a stretch is the ego." She teaches the jar theory of hip opening, which involves moving the pelvis in the opposite direction that the thigh bone moves. The theory is that you do not open a jar by turning the lid and the jar in the same direction. Jar theory and yoga theory agree that you have to go in two different directions for opening to occur.

Yoga is the practice of creating the conditions for opening to occur. One definition of yoga is the union of apparent opposites. If we just relate to mind, it's not yoga. If we just relate to body, it's not yoga. If we just relate to soft and flowing, or upbeat and happy, or love, love, love, we deny who we are. It is part of our humanness to feel anger, boredom, joy, agitation, elation, dullness, disappointment, and surprise. If we only allow ourselves to feel one way all the time we are not open, we are robots. Totally shut down and programmed.

As warriors we learn to face ourselves with a gentle heart that doesn't choose only some things to open to and others to reject. We learn to relax and open up to more feelings than just those that are comfortable or familiar. It doesn't mean we have to act out all our feelings, but we can watch them arise and pass as we stand firmly in warrior posture. This kind of fearlessness and opening allows us to begin to make friends with the variety of our own human repertoire of experiences, observe them with curiosity, and feel them even as they mutate into something else.

If we are one-dimensional, we cannot be open. If our mind gets hard in an effort to hold up our body, we are not open. It is only when we have the courage to stay open and awake to every moment, to flame the fire of burning enthusiasm just enough by applying precision and gentleness to our practice, that we can be warriors with open hearts and strong bodies.

NATURAL INTELLIGENCE

When people begin their yoga practice they are often self-conscious about the way their bodies look. Sometimes they tell me that they want to get in shape before they come to yoga class. I can assure you that as a yoga teacher I never look at students from a fashion viewpoint of "good body" or "bad body." I look at the flow of energy, the balance of strength and flexibility, of upper and lower body, movement of breath, tension in the face or voice. These are my cues for how I can help you, which is my honor and my job.

Most yogis arrive at this same perspective over time. When they feel a tight spot, or a dull spot, in their bodies, they don't have as much judgment as they once did. They tend to simply notice it and with curiosity begin to explore how they might be able to work with that situation, loosening it up, balancing it with movement on the other side, deepening the breath, using a prop such as a yoga block or bolster to help open muscles, breath, prana.

It's really no big deal. These issues are what we have to work with. If everything was pleasant all the time, and you could do every possible asana perfectly every time, you really wouldn't have anything to do in yoga class. Fatigued muscles, nagging story lines, buns that won't relax, these are what it means to be human. Take this opportunity to learn about yourself by watching your feelings, thoughts, and experiences—just like a flowing vinyasa—arise, hang out for a while, and then dissolve. Doing yoga is a good place to begin getting comfortable with this process because your body gives you a lot to work with in the form of immediate sensory feedback.

At the end of the day, yoga is not about how pretzel-like we can become or how long we can sit still. The actual practice is how we respond to sensory feedback—do we grasp it, push it away, ignore it? Start with applying precision to see what's what: "Ooh, my hamstring feels like it's been overstretched. Is the tender area at the top of the hamstring near the buttock or lower down by my knee?" Then gentleness: "I'm going to take my time getting warmed up today." Openness will help me to watch how this situation evolves without wallowing in self-judgment such as, "My yoga practice sucks because I can't even touch my toes." Now that I am armored with precise information, a gentle approach, and an open agenda, I can use my native intelligence to find the key for going forward: "What are some creative and beneficial modifications I can come up with for working with this injury?"

Our relationship with our body is a mirror of how we live our lives. Just like the rest of our life off the yoga mat and meditation cushion, we are always running into what seems like obstacles. How we deal with them is the practice. We can choose to try to conquer these challenges with a hard body and mind approach. But in the end, even if we solve the immediate problem we are still stuck with ourselves. Using a one-dimensional answer over and over will ultimately be unsatisfactory because we are not one-dimensional. Instead we can have the bravery to keep tuning in to what we feel—expansive, weak, burning, energized, sweaty—which is what keeps us present and awake and continues to remind us that rather than leading with our head, we can let it rest softly over our heart.

In *Shambhala: The Sacred Path of the Warrior,* Chögyam Trungpa Rinpoche writes, "The ideal of warriorship is that the warrior should be sad and tender, and because of that, the warrior can be very brave as well. Without that heartfelt sadness, bravery is brittle, like a china cup. If you drop it, it will break or chip. But the bravery of the warrior is like a lacquer cup, which has a wooden base covered with layers of lacquer. If the cup drops, it will bounce rather than break. It is soft and hard at the same time."

Cultivating this kind of multidimensional strength, inner and outer, focused and expansive, helps you connect to ahimsa, tapas, precision, gentleness, opening, and natural intelligence. Not too hard and not too soft, just the right ever-changing amounts of both. By having the courage to open to your own experience in an authentic and genuine way, you may find that the vibrancy of effort in your muscles, deepening in your breath, and heat in your belly are as much a part of you as the suppleness, joy, and maybe even peace of mind that accompany them.

YOGA BODY

STANDING ASANA SEQUENCES

Try to make a commitment to doing yoga on a regular basis. Do your practice even if you don't feel like it. This is where *tapas* comes in. Do only what is appropriate for you today. This is where *precision* comes in. You will know when you are doing that because you will be able to *gently* engage your body and mind fully, with the effort that that requires without getting hard-minded or hard-hearted. Stay *open* and watch what comes up for you.

Notice how your body feels as you do the following standing pose sequences, where you feel tight, slack, weak, bright, dull. At the same time, notice where your mind goes as your body feels these different things. Try to use your energy efficiently, so that you neither overexert yourself nor space out. Then don't worry about it. Use your bright awareness to observe how each time is different, how your body starts to get oiled up and opened up. You will see that what felt stressful yesterday now feels like a massage, and then how that good feeling vanishes but that's fine and no big deal. The next day you can take a fresh start. Watch how your mind and body find space again, which allows your breath to deepen and your mind to open even more. Without judgment, notice your mind chatter and with precision let it go. Doing this consistently will cultivate clarity, concentration, and confidence. This kind of commitment relates to the tapas of practice as well as the potential to experience enthusiasm for your ordinary life, which is richer than we could ever imagine.

BEGINNER STANDING SEQUENCE

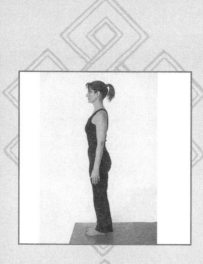

1. *Tadasana* • Mountain Pose

Take a moment to review the alignment principles of tadasana. Feel the earth supporting you and the sky above you. Let tadasana inform all your standing poses.

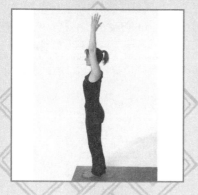

2. *Urdhva Hastasana* • Arms Up

inhale

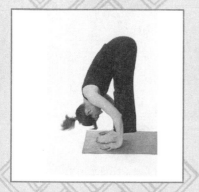

3. *Uttanasana 1* • Standing Forward Bend

exhale

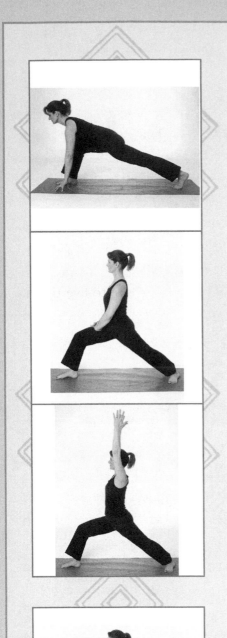

4. *Virabhadrasana 1* • Warrior 1

Step the left leg back into a low lunge and rise up on your fingertips. Take a moment here to lengthen your spine and strongly activate your left leg. Keeping the left leg energized, rotate the left heel toward the center of the mat, place your palms on your front thigh, and lift your spine up to a vertical position. Feel the broadness of your back and allow your front ribs and chest to soften back. If you feel strong enough, you can try lifting your arms up by your ears.

Remain in warrior 1 for a few breaths. You might find this quite challenging but try not to harden or hold the pose. Find the movement in it: the breath, your heartbeat, the tiny adjustments you might make to create openings or a deeper sense of grounding. Open your toes, your eyes, rest your mind.

5. *Virabhadrasana 2* • Warrior 2

On an exhale, open into warrior 2. Place one hand on the top of your head and one hand on your tailbone. Align these two points on a vertical axis, feel them reaching away from each other, and then extend your arms out from that midline. Can you still feel the strong centering of tadasana within this more expansive pose?

(The second time you come into warrior 2 on the other

side, try this exercise: Rotate your palms to face up to the ceiling. Can you feel how your shoulder blades move toward each other and are firm on your back? Maintain that external rotation in the upper arms but from the elbows to the fingertips internally rotate the arms so the palms face the floor. This is the same arm configuration that we use for almost all asanas. It opens the shoulders and balances the work of the arms.)

On an exhale, press your feet down into the ground and let that downward energy straighten your right leg. As you inhale, bend the right leg back into warrior 2. Repeat this little sequence, straightening and bending, three to five times. Feel how the exhale relates to downward-moving effort and the inhalation lifts the spine even as you are bending your right leg.

6. *Trikonasana* • Triangle Pose

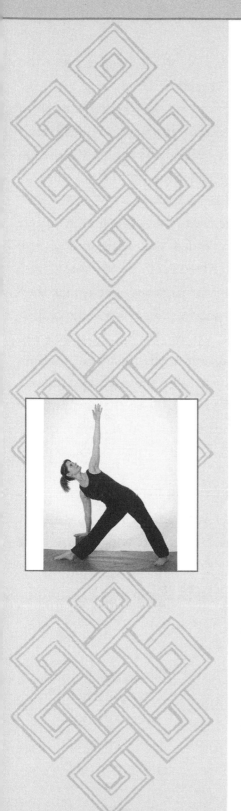

With straight legs, on an exhale, draw your right sitting bone under and toward your left inner thigh as you extend out through your spine in the opposite direction. Take a look at your right knee and make sure it is tracking directly over your right foot. If it means that you need to allow your left hip point to swing toward the right slightly, that is fine. Then, with the right leg in front, the pelvis rotates like a steering wheel making a right turn. It is not necessary for your pelvis to remain in an absolutely flat plane, but it is important for your knee to be in alignment with the foot.

Place your right hand on a block, or on your shin, moving into triangle pose. Find the place of extension without strain. Maintain grounding in the left foot. Soften the top ribs and lengthen the bottom ribs. Stay here for five breaths.

On an inhale, come back up to straight legs and exhale back into warrior 2.

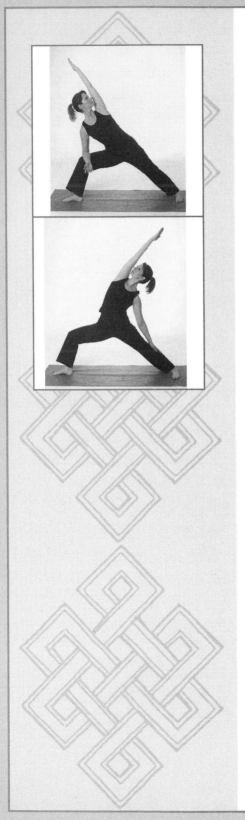

7. *Uttitha Parsvakonasana and Reverse Virabhadrasana 2* •
Extended Side Angle and Reverse Warrior

Exhale and place your right forearm on your right thigh in extended side angle. Inhale and reverse your side bend, lowering your left palm onto the outside of your left leg and extending your right arm up and over your right ear into reverse warrior.

Coordinating the movement with the breath, move back and forth between extended side angle and reverse warrior three to five times. Try to keep the legs strong and steady. This will challenge your right leg, but rather than coming out of the pose as soon as it gets intense, or just toughing it out, look for solutions. Explore how you can drop your weight into the center of the right foot, inviting the support of the right hamstring so the quadricep doesn't have to do all the work. This is one way that we practice extending the space between stimuli and response, which in turn offers us more options or solutions to challenging situations.

8. *Adho Mukha Svanasana* • Downward-Facing Dog

After your last reverse warrior, cartwheel your hands all the way down the floor on either side of the right leg and step into downward-facing dog. (Pictured on page 65.)

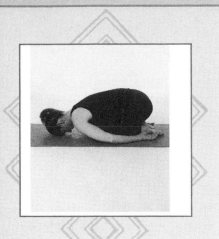

9. *Balasana* • Child's Pose
Take a rest in child's pose.

Repeat this entire sequence to this point with the left leg in front. Rest in child's pose. Back to downward-facing dog one more time.

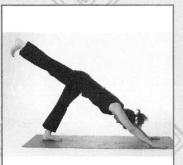

10. Downward-Facing Dog Split and Proposal Pose
On an inhale, lift your right leg up behind you in downward-facing dog split. Still thinking of tadasana, be mindful that your right leg stays in a parallel alignment, not rotating out as it might tend to do in this position.

As you exhale, swing your right foot forward and between your hands. Lower your left knee to the floor and organize your alignment so your legs are in a 90-degree arrangement. Inhale and lift your spine up to proposal pose.

Extend your left arm up and hook your right thumb in the outer crease of your right hip. This thumb will remind your hip not to ride up toward your right shoulder as you exhale and twist to the right.

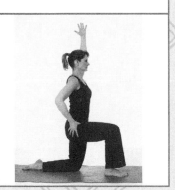

11. *Parivritta Parsvakonasana* • Rotated Side Angle Variation
Place your left elbow on the outside of your right knee and bring your hands together in anjali mudra, or prayer hands. As you inhale, think of lengthening the crown of the head and the tailbone away from each other. As you exhale, soften your belly and you might twist a little bit more. After five

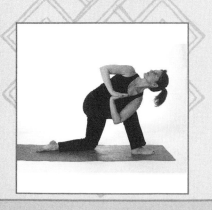

breaths, step back into downward-facing dog. (Pictured on page 65.)

Repeat the sequence (10-11) to the other side.

12. *Tadasana* • Mountain Pose
From downward-facing dog slowly walk your feet up to your hands. Think of this as a walking meditation. It's fine if you have to bend your knees along the way. When you are folded in half, place your palms on the top of your buttock flesh, as if you were putting your hands in the back pockets of your blue jeans. Press the buttock flesh down and let the action lift you back up to standing in tadasana. (Pictured on page 67.)

INTERMEDIATE STANDING SEQUENCE
Begin by doing the first six asanas of the intermediate sun salute:

1. *Tadasana* • Mountain Pose
(Pictured on page 67.)

2. *Urdhva Hastasana* • Arms Up
inhale
(Pictured on page 67.)

3. Swan Dive into Uttanasana 1
exhale
(Pictured on page 67.)

4. *Uttanasana 2* • Forward Bend with Long Spine
inhale
(Pictured on page 77.)

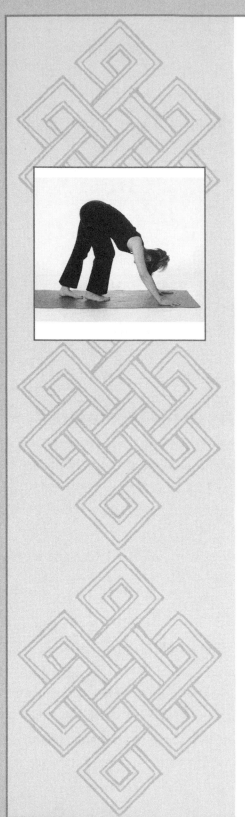

5. Jump Back

exhale

(Pictured on page 74.)

6. *Adho Mukha Svanasana* • Downward-Facing Dog

exhale

(Pictured on page 65.)

(Note: Photos are shown for second side with left leg forward.)

7. *Virabhadrasana 1* • Warrior 1

inhale

Turn your left heel to the floor, inhale and lift your spine and arms up. This time press your palms together. Let this be your warrior's sword that cuts through your story line.

Try to maintain length in the back of the neck. Can you lift your back inner ankle so the inner left leg is supported? You might feel the beginning of a backbending action in the lengthening of the front left hip.

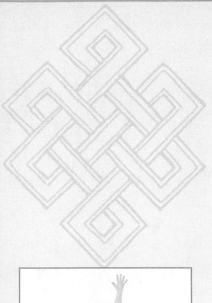

8. *Virabhadrasana 2* • Warrior 2

exhale

Exhale and expand into the vastness of warrior 2. Can you let the warrior's sword of your arms open up your heart to what is happening right now?

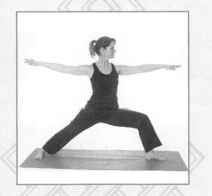

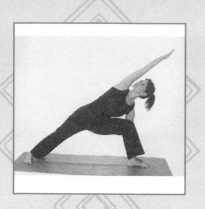

9. *Uttitha Parsvakonasana* • Extended Side Angle

Look for evenness in both sides of the ribs. Keep the collarbones broad and find the support of the shoulder blades on the back. Imagine the space underneath your legs supporting you like a big firm pillow of air. Stay here for five to eight breaths.

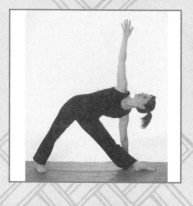

10. *Trikonasana* • Triangle Pose

You can keep your hand where it is or you might want to move it onto your shin or a block. As you exhale, press your right foot into the ground and draw your right sitting bone back toward your left inner thigh, moving into triangle. Extend the top arm up and feel your middle fingers reaching away from each other. Let both legs be equally active. Let both sides of the ribs be equally mobile, as you watch your breath going out and going in. Five to eight breaths.

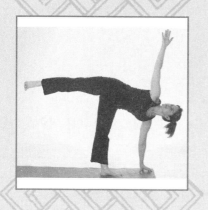

11. *Ardha Chandrasana* • Half Moon

Walk your right hand out about ten inches away from your right foot and place your left hand on your left waist. On an inhale, lift your left leg up as you extend your head in the opposite direction, feeling long. Make sure that your standing leg stays parallel and does not begin to rotate in, which is common in this pose. You can check this by seeing if your toes are in the same placement they were in triangle or if they have gone pigeontoed. Liberate your left arm up to the ceiling and extend out through all your limbs. Stay here for five to eight breaths.

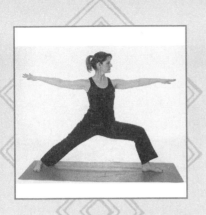

12. *Virabhadrasana 2* • Warrior 2

exhale

Gracefully float back down to warrior 2. This is hard to do but the trying can be fun. Try working like this: Reach the left heel and your right knee away from each other and drop your pelvis right in between them as you lift your spine up to warrior 2. All the actions and intentions have to happen together and it's a lot to wrap your mind around. My recommendation is to relax your mind and fly.

13. Reverse Warrior

inhale

As soon as you arrive back in warrior 2, let your inhale lift you into reverse warrior for one big breath.

Continue almost to the end of surya namaskar by cartwheeling your hands to the floor and going right down into chaturanga, all on one exhalation.

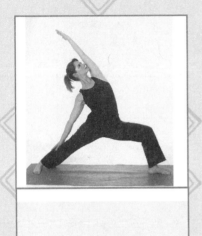

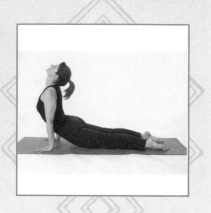

14. *Urdhva Mukha Svanasana* • Upward-Facing Dog
inhale

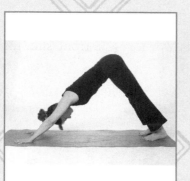

15. *Adho Mukha Svanasana* • Downward-Facing Dog
exhale
Stay here for three full breaths.

Repeat entire sequence 1–15 on other side.

16. End of Surya Namaskar
On the last exhale, bend your knees, look at the space between your hands, and jump there. Upon arrival, inhale to uttanasana 2 (Forward Bend with Long Spine). As you exhale, fold over to uttanasana 1.

17. *Utkatasana* • Powerful Pose
From uttanasana 1, instead of reversing the swan dive, bend your knees and lift your arms and spine into what is sometimes called awkward pose. What do you need to do to not feel awkward here? If your back is strained, straighten your legs a bit. If your chest or throat are tight, separate your arms. Feel smoothness and breath all around your neck and throat, as if you were wearing an evenly strung skin necklace.

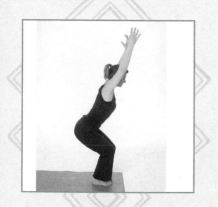

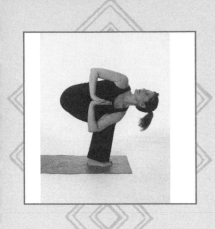

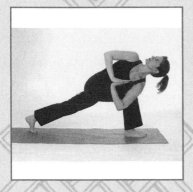

Find the fun in this pose by reaching your sitting bones way back as if you were being seated at an elegant dinner table and your date didn't push the chair in enough. Stay here for five breaths. What's happening in your mind here? What if you had to do this pose for twenty-five breaths?

On an inhale, lower your hands in front of your heart in anjali mudra. As you exhale, twist to the right, bringing your left elbow on the outside of your right knee.

18. *Parivritta Parsvakonasana* • Rotated Side Angle

Keep your eyes on your front foot. Move the front shin forward as you step your left leg back into a lunge. If the two legs energize away from each other evenly, your pelvis will feel light and balanced. Stay here for five breaths.

Step your left leg forward on an exhale, and untwist back into utkatasana.

19. *Virabhadrasana 1* • Warrior 1

Keeping your arms and your left leg in utkatasana, step your right leg back into warrior 1. (Pictured on page 101.)

Exhale to straighten your front leg. Extend your arms out to the sides and internally rotate them. Bring your palms together in anjali mudra behind your back. A prayer to hold up your heart from behind. If this is not possible for you today, try it with the fingers pointing down, or you can hold on to opposite wrists or elbows. Check your alignment here and make sure that the hands behind your back are not popping your front ribs forward.

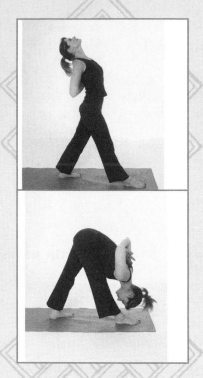

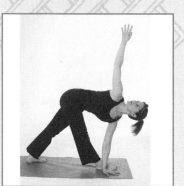

20. *Parsvottanasana* • Side Stretch

Inhale and lift your chest and face up to the ceiling, still dropping the tailbone down to the floor. Exhale, deepen the groins, and fold over your legs. You may feel a lot of sensation in the front hamstrings but be sure to keep grounding in the back heel to balance the work of both legs. Touching your nose to your leg is not that thrilling after the first few times, so try to relax those kinds of short-term goals and just see what is what.

This is called side stretch. What opening can you discover, especially in the upper ribs below the armpits? Try to keep your collarbones wide apart so your shoulders don't curl forward and smush your heart.

Stay here for five to eight breaths.

21. *Parivritta Trikonasana* • Rotated Triangle

Release your arms and inhale your spine parallel to the floor. Place your left hand on the outside of your right foot. You may wish to use a block or lift up onto your fingers, making a shape with your hands like the claw of an old-fashioned bathtub.

You can explore different feet alignments by drawing a line between the heels: they can be over crossed slightly with the front heel dissecting the back arch, which is most challenging and sometimes causes stress on the lower back; the heels can be in line with each other; or the back heel can be over the side slightly, which you may find easiest for learning this pose.

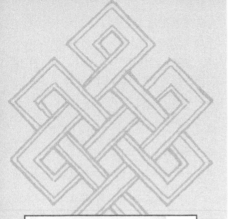

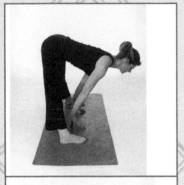

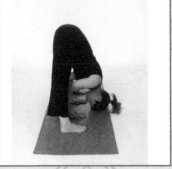

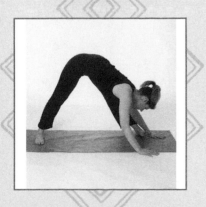

This is like being on a tightrope so don't worry about it if you fall over while you are learning this pose. Looking at your front foot will give you a landmark for where your spine is and then you can try to rotate around that axis. Reach down with the ball of your front big toe and draw up diagonally with your outer hip crease. Stay here for five to eight breaths.

22. *Prasarita Padottanasana* • Extended Legs Forward Bend
Exhale and untwist out of rotated triangle. Fold over your front leg and begin to walk your hands around to the left as you parallel your feet. Place your fingertips in line with your toe tips and inhale to a flat back position here. As you exhale, bend your elbows straight back like in chaturanga and lightly place the top of your head on the floor. If it doesn't touch the floor today, you can separate your feet a little bit more, or you can place a block under your head.

Here's another chance to pay attention to your situation as it is and make appropriate choices. Let your warrior's mind and heart cut through any craving thoughts. Straining won't help, so relax your spine, shoulders, and arms. But do keep your legs activated, muscles moving up the bones, just like in tadasana. Five to eight breaths.

23. End of Sequence
Walk yourself over to the left leg, lift your right heel, and step into downward-facing dog (pictured on page 104). Stay here for three full breaths and on the last exhale, jump forward. Complete the end of the surya namaskar series, ending back in utkatasana.

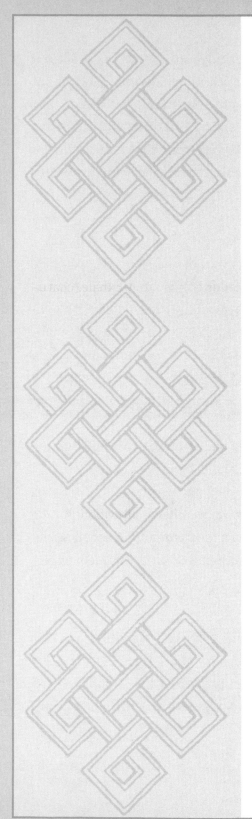

Repeat this sequence (17-23) to the other side and then stand up, back in tadasana right where you began.

ADVANCED STANDING SEQUENCE
Begin with the first seven poses of the advanced sun salute:

1. *Tadasana* • Mountain Pose
(Pictured on page 67.)

2. *Urdhva Hastasana* • Arms Up
inhale
(Pictured on page 67.)

3. Swan Dive into Uttanasana 1
exhale
(Pictured on page 67.)

4. *Uttanasana 2* • Forward Bend with Long Spine
inhale
(Pictured on page 77.)

5. Jump Back into Chaturanga Dandasana
exhale
(Pictured on page 79.)

6. *Urdhva Mukha Svanasana* • Upward-Facing Dog
inhale
(Pictured on page 75.)

7. *Adho Mukha Svanasana* • Downward-Facing Dog
exhale
(Pictured on page 76.)

8. *Virabhadrasana 1 and 2* • Warrior 1 and 2
Exhale and turn your left heel down, step your right foot behind your hands. Inhale up to warrior 1. Exhale and open to warrior 2. (Pictured on page 101.)

9. Advanced Vinyasa Flow
Inhale and cartwheel your hands to the floor. Exhale, chaturanga, inhale, upward-facing dog, exhale, downward-facing dog. (Pictured on page 104.)

Repeat warrior 1, warrior 2, and the vinyasa flow to the other side.

Repeat again right and left, two more times each side, ending in downward-facing dog. (Pictured on page 104.)

The following sequence is a development of the intermediate sequence so you can do that one first to prepare.

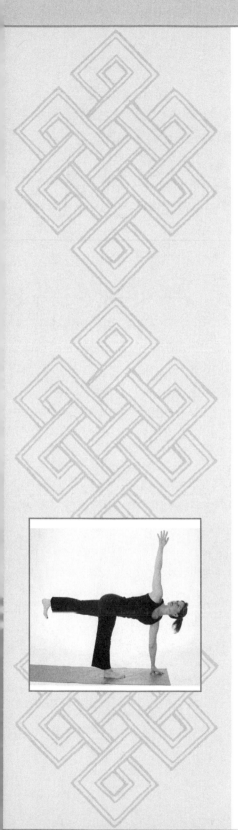

10. *Parivritta Ardha Chandrasana* • Rotated Half Moon
Step your right leg forward into a lunge. Place your right fingers in your right outer hip crease and walk your left fingertips forward on the floor about eight inches in front of your foot. Inhale and lift your left leg up behind, keeping it parallel in a downward-facing doglike position. On the exhale begin to twist to the right. Keep your fingers in your right hip until you are fully twisted, then extend the arm up to the ceiling.

Cartwheel your right arm down, left arm up, and step your left leg back to arrive in warrior 2. This is a fun transition and the way to manage it is to keep equal awareness in

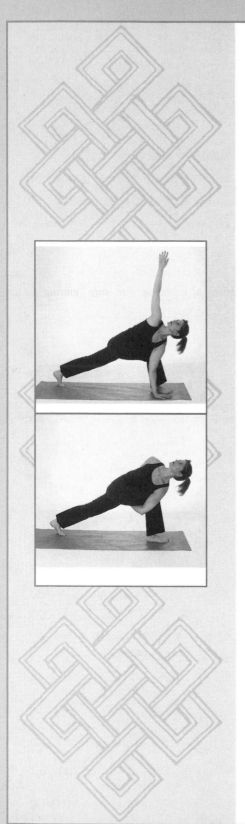

both arms, legs, and spine. Letting go in all directions in order to find stability in your center.

Lift your back heel and spin your chest around to move into a high lunge with the arms up.

The next three poses will be a good opportunity to apply precision, without aggression, and a chance to try new challenges with an open mind.

11. *Parivritta Parsvakonasana* • Rotated Side Angle

On an exhale, twist to the right. Place your left upper arm on the outside of your right leg, being mindful to keep your right knee tracking directly forward. Sometimes if your back is tight, the twist available to you isn't deep enough to allow your arm to go outside your leg and that will pull the knee off its strong and safe position. If that is the case, place your hand on a block, or put your hands in anjali mudra, as in the intermediate version of the twist in utkatasana. Either way, you can then extend the top arm up. Keeping the back leg active will help you to anchor this pose.

If you feel balanced and can breathe fully in this pose, then feel free to continue with this sequence. Internally rotate your top arm and bring it around behind your back. Internally rotate your bottom arm and slip it under your right thigh. Even though it seems counterintuitive, if you reach your left fingers toward the back of your right knee you will find your right fingertips over time. Be sure to keep twisting to the right and opening the right armpit chest area. You may be able to make a bind, with the left hand holding the right wrist.

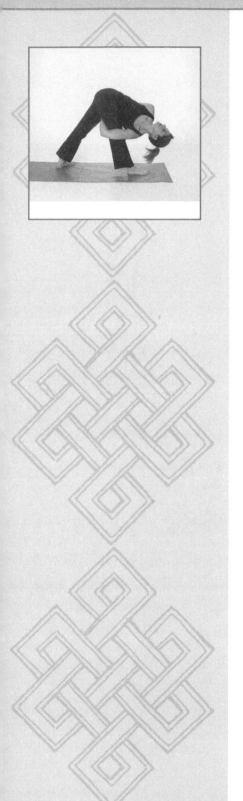

12. *Baddha Parivritta Trikonasana* • Bound Rotated Triangle
From the bound variation of rotated side angle, step your back leg in slightly, turn the heel down as if you were in warrior 1, and lengthen your front leg. Draw the right hip back and spin the left ribs under. It is a challenge to breathe here, maintain balance, create opening in the lower back and shoulders, and still feel spacious. What is your experience?

Release out of this pose and step back into downward-facing dog. (Pictured on page 104).

Take a rest in child's pose and then try the other side, ending in downward-facing dog (steps 10-12).

Complete the sequence by jumping forward and finishing the rest of the advanced sun salute (pages 79-80).

SEVEN

DYNAMIC EQUANIMITY

Balancing Poses

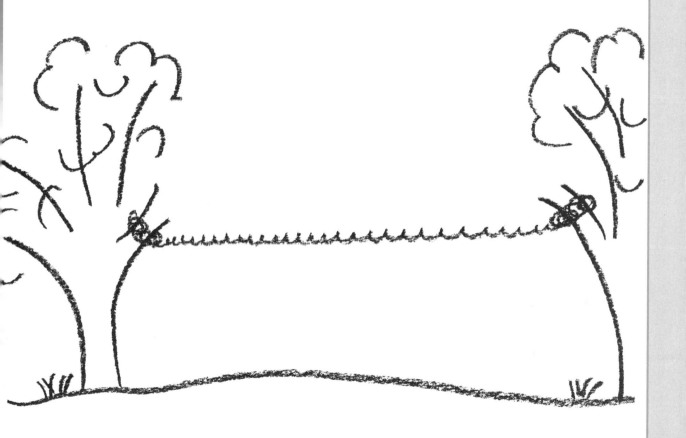

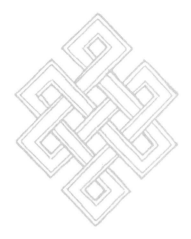

Yoga Body

What do the following things have in common: riding a bike with no hands, trees, marriage, sailing a boat, yoga, walking a tightrope, a set of scales, circus performers, the stock market?

They are all about finding balance in a highly mobile situation. The list is endless and could pretty much include everything in life. That understanding is the key to our yoga and meditation practice. Balance comes from the Latin word *balare,* which means to dance. Rather than looking to establish a solid state of bliss that never shifts (like a sunny day that lasts forever), we are looking for a means of dancing with our world as it moves, a way of feeling the richness of both joy and sadness, of watching with curiosity as the weather changes.

We know that our mind and body are really one, they're both us, right? Then when our physicality is balanced, so is our mind, translating into a sense of well-being and confidence. Practicing meditation, which helps us watch our mind-movies without judgment, and yoga, which develops our strong and flexible body, are the means to an end. The end, which is, of course, without end, is to live a balanced life.

An anchored sailboat is a perfect example of dynamic equanimity. There is simply no such thing as stationary balance. If something was completely unmoving it would be unnatural, out of balance. Sometimes people think yoga is about changing your religion, your eating habits, or the way you dress. But whatever changes you might make will not bring you a balanced experience if they remain fixed. A new religion, a food dogma, any point of view that is rigid leads to fundamentalism, which is a very quick way to shut yourself off from the world. Our practice is an opportunity to stay open to every new situation, and stay on point, sailing the middle path, by relating appropriately to how the wind is blowing that very minute.

The only ingredients we can rely on to experience balance are our own body, speech or breath, and mind. We like to think that we can lean on our external situations—the house, a job, our children—as if they were unchanging. But none of those elements are fixed entities, and when we grasp at them for security, we lose the opportunity for a balanced life. The kids will grow up and leave; you may get downsized at work; and your plumbing—both in your house and in your body—can spring a leak without warning. Nothing is solid. Even the planet we live on is hurling through space. Rather than going through life on automatic pilot, counting on everything staying the same, and then getting hit with surprises that throw us topsy-turvy, by familiarizing ourselves with the rhythms of our own body, breath, and mind, we can learn how to sail through our life, no matter what the weather report.

MOVEMENT OF THE BODY

The first step to experiencing balance in the body is by grounding down into the earth. Establish your "seat" in each asana. What part of your body is touching the ground? What part of your body is moving earthward right now?

If you live in a big city like I do, touching the actual ground is a rare experience. In June 2001, I taught a short yoga class to a crowd of over a thousand meditators who had come to New York's Central Park for *Tricycle* magazine's annual Change Your Mind day. I was so accustomed to teaching indoors that I kept guiding the crowd of yogis to press their feet firmly into the floor and extend their arms up to the ceiling, even though we were outside. It is important for all of us to actually feel dirt and grass and earth as often as possible, to be able to have that tangible memory of connection to the life-giving energy of the earth. We cannot truly be grounded without surrendering to this support. The energy of this downward yielding will organically rebound and begin to lift our spine and upper body, creating both stability and liberation.

On the physical plane, we tend to think of balance as something stationary and unmoving. Standing on one leg and holding tree pose for three breaths is certainly an accomplishment, but if simply holding a shape is the extent of our experience of balance, we will feel more like a rock than a tree. Once we have our grounding, the next step is to allow movement to happen.

Try this. Stand in tadasana with your feet firmly planted on the floor and your arms down by your sides. Close your eyes. Don't do anything. Just stand there. You will soon begin to notice quite a lot of movement within the stillness of simply standing. You will feel the movement of your body, expanding and contracting as you breathe, you will feel the pulse of your own heartbeat, you will feel your entire body swaying slightly in order to stay balanced on this big round ball we live on. In fact, if you were truly static, the earth's movement would eventually tip you over. Can you relax and let your body do this dance of balance?

Julia Butterfly Hill discovered how to do this during her two-year residency in Luna, a thousand-year-old redwood tree in northern California. Julia was committed to living in the treetop for as long as it took to convince the Pacific Lumber Company to stop destroying old-growth forests and causing disastrous environmental problems throughout the region. In early 1998, more than sixty days since she had touched the earth with her own two feet, she heard radio warnings of seventy-mile-per-hour storm winds coming her way. Her survival instincts told her to climb down, but she was afraid that if she left Luna, the tree would be cut down. She recounts her experience in her book *The Legacy of Luna*:

I was trying to hold onto life so hard that my teeth were clenched, my fists were clenched, everything in my body was clenched completely and totally tight. . . . I knew I was going to die. . . . Had I remained tensed for the sixteen hours that the storm raged, I would have snapped. Instead . . . as I started to picture the trees in the storm, the answer began to dawn on me.

The trees in the storm don't try to stand up straight and tall and erect. They allow themselves to bend and be blown with the wind. They understand the power of letting go. . . . Those trees and those branches that try too hard to stand up strong and straight are the ones that break. . . . Learn the power of the trees. Let it flow. Let it go. That is the way you are going to make it through this storm. And that is the way to make it through the storms of life.

Julia Butterfly Hill's strong commitment ultimately became the ground for freedom and transformation, for both herself and Luna. From this kind of rooting down, we can also be like trees and let our upper bodies move with freedom. But how do we both hold a shape and allow for movement to happen? By connecting to the experiencing of motion and change, just as Julia did, rather than fixing on how something *should* be or feel, or what a shape *should* look like.

People ask me all the time what they should feel in this pose or that pose. Although each asana is very precise in how it activates certain muscle groups, heats up and purifies inner organs, and creates specific energetic circuits that affect the nervous system in beneficial ways, I do not know what you should be feeling. I can tell you whether your body is aligned properly, or if you are overworking one area of the body. I can point out when your attention is too intense or too wild, and let you know when you are placing yourself in a potentially injurious position, but I cannot tell you what your own experience should be, except that it should be completely personal to you.

Many people prefer to be told what they should think or feel or believe, but yoga and meditation don't do that for you—and a good teacher won't do that for you either. We've all heard, "No pain, no gain." Some people think that if they don't feel anything intensely they aren't getting the benefit of the pose. But if you are alive, there is no way you are not feeling something. It takes being quiet, paying attention, and opening to movement to find out what we are feeling. If we don't know how we felt in the first place how do we know if we are feeling any different, if anything even happened? Practice will reveal this process to you. It will expose what you already think and feel and believe. Recognizing your own fixations, and how they are holding you back from living as full a life as possible, is the first step to letting go and opening to movement, space, possibility.

Challenge yourself to approach your life with an open agenda. Let your balancing asanas be a way to practice that. A sailing captain has a big bag of tricks based on training, maps, computerized compasses, experience, and intuition, but he does not know what the wind and water are going to be like that day. Try not to put on your tree pose like you were putting on a coat. If you wear an asana the same way you wore it yesterday, you will notice that it no longer fits. Let go of the craving to accomplish any of these balancing positions and see where they take you today.

MOVEMENT OF THE BREATH

One of the most easily accessible forms of energy moving through our body is our wind energy or breathing. The quality of the breath is in direct relationship to both the experience of the mind and the condition of the body. When we become disturbed by external circumstances, our breathing pattern changes. We may gasp, sigh, hold our breath, or even scream, which is an exhale. This breathing response will, in turn, intensify our already unbalanced emotional state, causing it to be even more agitated. This kind of zigzag recycling of reactions creates a bottleneck of energy. *Pranayama* is sometimes translated as "to release life energy from its bounds," and it's true that when we can free the breath from both mental and physical constraints, it's as good as opening a tight belt after Thanksgiving dinner.

Pranayama is, first of all, a form of familiarization. It is an elemental way of knowing who we are, on all levels—heart, body, and mind. Patanjali's Yoga Sutra says the practice of pranayama "removes the veil from the light of consciousness." Pranayama is a practice of learning about ourselves through learning about our breath, about cultivating a new relationship to the breath, and about learning to recognize what is called our authentic breath. Over time the practice of breath awareness will begin to reverse the habitual breathing tendency of emotion breathing affecting emotion in a downward spiral, as the authentic breath begins to simply "happen" naturally in our practice and in our everyday lives.

When you practice balancing poses, notice your breathing tendencies. Your breath may be stormlike or it may be gentle. Understand your breath rather than invent a certain manner of breathing. Often students try to make their breath get loud, like Darth Vader, possibly in an unconscious attempt to create something to hold on to. Your breath can be like a life raft that rescues you but only if you jump on as it floats by. If you grab on it, then it stops floating, causing you to drown or suffocate.

There is no right or wrong way for each breath to feel. Every breath is different, like fingerprints and snowflakes. Notice when you feel off balance and what happens to your breath in that moment. Did you hold, harden, or grab your breath? Can you reverse the pattern? Explore the possibility of maintaining a smooth breathing pattern, in and out, equally through your whole body, as a fluid support for balance.

Observe the movement of the breath throughout your entire body. Even though you know you are breathing in and out with your nose and the air is going into your lungs, the exchange of oxygen and carbon dioxide is happening throughout your bloodstream, so in reality, you are breathing with every cell in your body. Soften your mind so you can experience this three-dimensional expansion and contraction. As you connect to this oscillation, you may be able to feel this motion in your pose, too. Imagine that your balancing pose is an anchored sailboat and your breath is the water. Let the breath gently move the pose so that it is alive.

BUDDHA MIND

MOVEMENT OF THE MIND

You may have already discovered that yoga gives you a tool bag full of goodies such as patience, compassion, curiosity, and nonjudging that help you navigate the ups and downs of life. After doing yoga for even a short while, people tell me things like "My husband says I'm easier to live with." "I'm nicer to waiters." "I don't get so upset in traffic." This is the beginning of deep composure or equanimity. The path to equanimity is not being attached to the fruits of your actions.

On September 5, 1978, I moved to New York City with Michael Holly, my boyfriend at that time. We visited Washington Square Park the first day we arrived. We were excited by the folk singers, comedians, disco-rollers, and other street performers in the park. But when we came upon a tightrope walker in a top hat and tuxedo, Michael became transfixed. The next day he decided to teach himself to walk a tightrope and to juggle. He bought a rope, a winch, and a bag of colored rubber balls. Michael picked out two good trees in Central Park, hooked up the rope three feet off the ground, jumped up, and got started.

He was extremely disciplined in practicing these two skills. Sometimes when I sat in our little Greenwich Village studio apartment watching rubber balls flying at lamps, dishes, and the TV, I thought he was obsessed. But it was fun for him. He didn't have a booking he was working toward, or an agent who was egging him on, or any goal whatsoever except to see if he could figure out how to walk on a tightrope and juggle, possibly at the same time. He learned that he should wear slippers instead of sneakers, and that bean bags were more forgiving than balls that roll away.

Looking back, I see now that Michael did two things right. First, he didn't care how long it took for him to master these skills. That approach made it impossible for him to fail, so he was never tempted to give up, even on those days when he felt off-kilter and uncoordinated.

Second, he didn't care if he fell off the rope. I never saw him get frustrated about that. He would just lose his balance, fall off, and get back on. No big deal. Even when he started working with a higher rope, he taught himself to catch it when he fell and hoist himself back up without ever touching the ground. He was very practical. He wanted to learn these two things so he created an open agenda that would support his exploration. That freedom made it fun for him and so his discipline was never a chore. Eventually he figured out pretty much everything about walking on a rope as well as juggling anything from bowling balls to M&Ms, and today, Michael has a successful act as a juggling comedian in Las Vegas.

Michael was not attached to the fruits of his action, and because of that, he was able to be in balance, to experience equanimity. Equanimity is not something that can be accomplished or finished, but, like yoga and meditation, it is a process. Equanimity, balance, is the essence of yoga. It is a liminal state of neither in nor out, but both at once. When you are standing in a doorway, you know you can choose the future or the past, forward or back, open or closed, but once you leave that threshold you have chosen just that one thing.

Riding balance, being on the threshold of a doorway, does not require making a fixed choice, but allows us to be more than one thing. When we explore balance, we are expanding our options. This is yoga—finding the relationship between apparent opposites. We all have a tendency to want things to be clear—in or out, good or bad, half empty or half full—and we get nervous when things are in a gray area. But everything is always shades of gray because everything is in constant fluctuation, like the sailboat and the tree. Learning to ride the movement of balance is a way to gain the confidence to make new choices, to expand the choices, to learn how to rest in the gray areas.

Life doesn't always unfold the way we plan. If we don't allow ourselves to connect to the dance of our relationships, traffic, and the unfolding of life, moment to moment, not only do we miss opportunities but we become profoundly uncomfortable. This is how we create our own suffering. The beauty of yoga and meditation is that you cannot get it wrong. Yoga and meditation are not about mastering a body of knowledge, but about becoming familiar with our state of mind. It is a repetitive process that at first leads to boredom and irritation and then gets very, very interesting.

This is challenging and takes time—and practice! If you think of balance as a motorcycle, you could think of patience as the sidecar. You cannot rush and be balanced. Fortunately, cultivating patience is easy. All you have to do is wait. At my first fourteen-day meditation retreat our teacher told us that our practice was about "resting in a state of not-knowing." He also helped us by saying that this kind of composure takes a long time to develop. It takes patience to develop patience.

Michael was patient because he didn't have a finish line in the front of his mind. He was more interested in what might happen today. In our own way we can all do the same thing Michael did when he created an environment for himself that supported exploration, discovery, and possibility.

Falling is simply part of the process of learning to balance. Every baby knows this. If they stopped trying every time they fell, none of us would be walking today. Being on balance and falling are two sides of the same coin. The way to experiencing a balanced life includes falling, dusting ourselves off, looking at what we learned from that experience, and getting back on the program. My teacher, Gehlek Rimpoche, explains it this way:

"How does spiritual development grow within a person? It is not going to suddenly hit you. It only works this way—you go and go and fall and get up and move and go and fall. Fall down on your face, get up, clean it up, remove, wash it, put your dust off, go and you fall down. Doesn't matter, get up, go. Falling down doesn't matter, get up; fall down—that doesn't matter, get up again. Get up a hundred thousand times. That is what it really is. Nobody is perfect. Nobody can do it right from the beginning. Everybody, including Buddha, went that way: fall down, get up, fall down, get up. And that is what we should do. And if when fallen down twice or three times, you say, "Ah, forget about it," it is worse; that is really bad, very bad. That is shutting down your own development, totally shutting it, like shutting the door. Fall, get up, move, fall, get up, move! Everybody does, it doesn't matter, don't feel bad, but feel happy about it, go ahead. That is how people move, otherwise everybody should be a Buddha from the beginning. No, nobody is. So don't even worry when you fall down; it doesn't matter, but make sure you get up! That is very important. If you fall down and you sit there, you remain there. Make sure you get up. That's what it is."

Enjoy falling, it's your most valuable tool for learning balancing poses. When you fall you learn about how much effort to use, how to stack your bones, how to use your visual focus, how to ride on the movement of the breath. You will still be developing strength and flexibility, coordination, and stamina whether you stay in the pose or fall out. The actual pose is not going to get you through your day but the composure, equanimity, balance, and patience that arises from standing on the threshold of every moment will.

YOGA BODY

BALANCING ASANA SEQUENCES

The following sequences explore balance in many dimensions: one arm and one leg, two arms and one leg, sitting bones only, arms only, front and back, effort and release, intention and surprise. As you do your balancing asana sequences, remember to establish your seat first. What part of you is touching the earth? Then begin to observe your breath and let it give you feedback about if and where you are trying to make your pose solid—gripping with your eyes, your calves, your tummy. Rest in a state of not-knowing by allowing the movement of the breath, the earth, your heartbeat, all to contribute to the fresh experience of your practice today.

BEGINNER BALANCING SEQUENCE, OR WARM-UP VINYASA

Every action gets one breath, but at first you might wish to go slower and explore the balance and movement of each position.

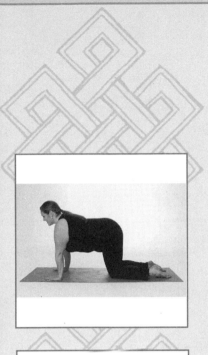

Hands and Knees
Make sure your wrists are directly below your shoulders and your knees are below your hips.

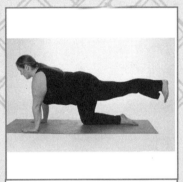

On an *inhale,* extend your right leg behind you and off the floor. Look slightly forward and lightly tone your belly.

    Exhale and replace your leg to the floor.

Inhale as you lift your left leg up behind you. Reach out evenly through all four corners of the foot.

    Exhale and replace the foot to the floor.

Inhale and lift the right leg up again but this time add the left arm, too.

    Exhale, leg and arm back down.

    Repeat to the other side.

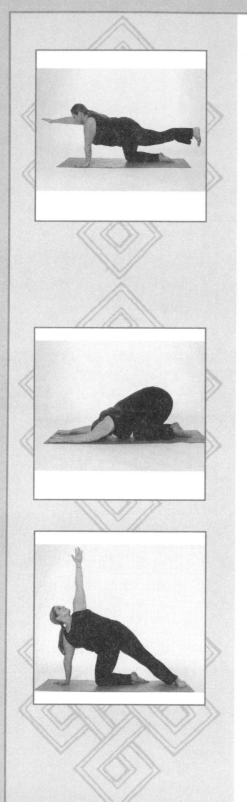

Inhale and lift the right leg up one more time but this time add the right arm—same arm and leg. Just see what it feels like and don't worry about falling. In this position, it's not that far down to the floor.

Exhale, replace your arm and leg to the floor.

Do the other side, too.

Inhale the right leg back behind you but stay in contact with the floor. Turn your right heel down and shift your weight onto your left hand.

Exhale as you spin your belly to the right and reach your right arm up.

Inhale back to hands and knees.

Exhale into child's pose.

Inhale right back to hands and knees and extend your left leg back all in one deep breath.

Exhale rotating to the left, left arm up.

Inhale back to hands and knees.

Exhale into child's pose.

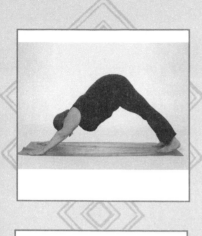

Inhale once again to hands and knees.

   Exhale as you press your hips up into downward-facing dog.

Inhale to reach your right hand around behind you and touch your right sitting bone.

   Exhale and replace your right hand down.

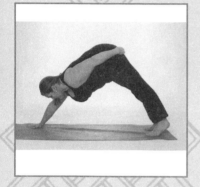

Inhale and touch your left sitting bone with your left hand.

   Exhale your left hand back down. (Are you sure those are your sitting bones? They are the little walnutlike bones that you actually sit on. Their anatomical name is ischial tuberosities, which always reminds me of tubers so I think of our sitting bones as the root vegetables of our bodies.)

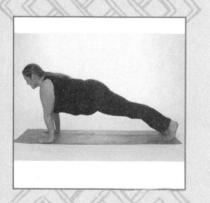

Inhale moving into plank pose. Have a sense of the armpits and sternum reaching forward as the heels extend back.

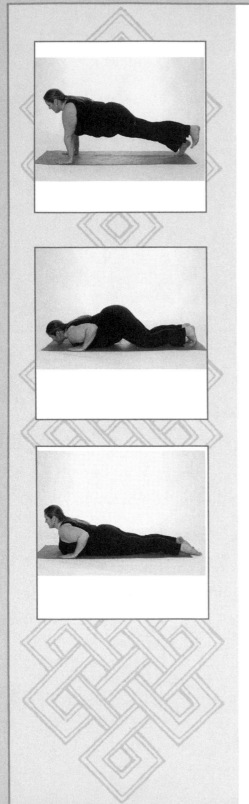

Exhale as you lift your right foot off the floor just two tiny inches.

Inhale and replace your foot to the floor.
    Exhale the other leg up.
    Inhale as you lightly place it back down.

Exhale, lower knees, chest, and chin to the floor.

Inhale to baby cobra.

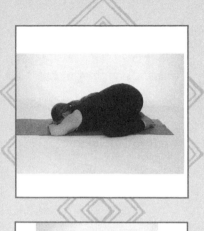

Exhale and press back into child's pose. Rest here for a few breaths.

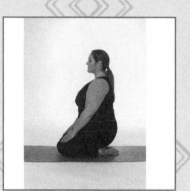

Inhale to lift you up to vajrasana.

Repeat this entire sequence.

INTERMEDIATE BALANCING SEQUENCE

Begin with surya namaskar, moving through to the first downward-facing dog.

1. *Vasisthasana* • Side Inclined Plane

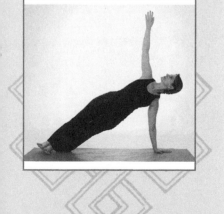

Shift your weight onto your left hand and left leg. Draw your tailbone forward as you find your balance in vasisthasana. This is how you would look if you were standing in tadasana and a big wind blew you over. It's not just about arm strength. Use your legs just as much as if you were standing on your two feet.

Now, be brave and lift your right leg up off the left leg two inches. Keep both legs active, extending through the four cor-

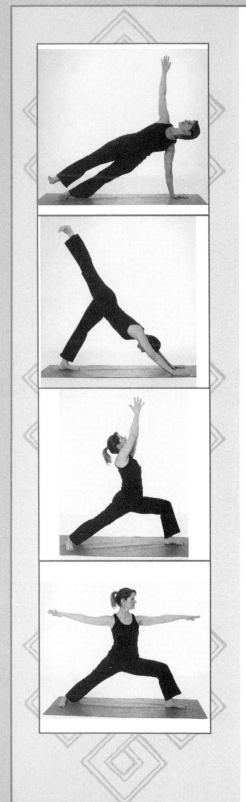

ners of both feet. Keep your right leg airborne and shift your hips right over into downward-facing dog split.

Take a big breath in and as you exhale, swing your right leg all the way through your hands.

Inhale up to virabhadrasana 1 (warrior 1).

Exhale open to virabhadrasana 2 (warrior 2).

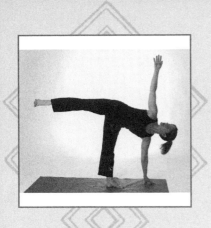

2. *Ardha Chandrasana* • Half Moon

Inhale into ardha chandrasana and stay here for a few breaths. Feel the relationship between your pubic bone and tailbone, front and back ribs, right and left fingers, crown of the head and back heel. See what happens if you turn your head to look up. If you go too fast or throw your head back you might fall over. Think of simply placing your right ear under your left ear. Remember your neck is an extension of your spine. Can you feel the conversation between the sky that you are seeing and the earth that you are feeling?

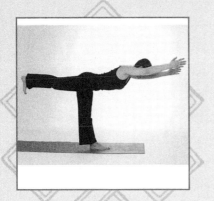

3. *Virabhadrasana 3* • Warrior 3

Exhale and rotate your pelvis so both hip points face the floor. Extend both arms forward and feel the space underneath you holding you up. Stay here for three breaths.

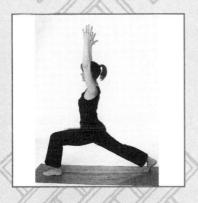

On an inhale, move the front shin and the back heel away from each other, gracefully arriving in a high lunge.

Exhale, chaturanga dandasana (four-limbed stick pose). (Pictured on page 79.)

Inhale, urdhva mukha svanasana (upward-facing dog). (Pictured on page 103.)

Exhale, adho mukha svanasana (downward-facing dog). (Pictured on page 104.)

Repeat this sequence beginning with vasisthasana on the right hand and right foot and ending back in downward-facing dog.

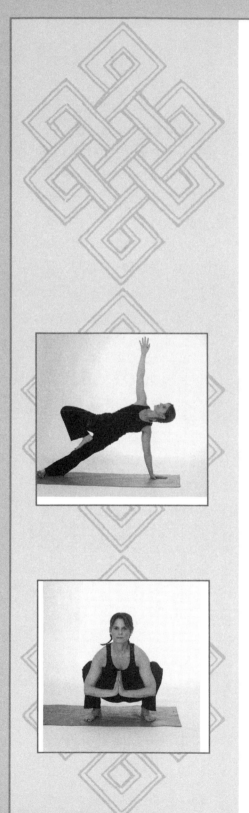

4. *Vasisthasana Variation* • Side Inclined Plane with Tree Pose
From downward-facing dog, shift into vasisthasana on the left hand and left foot again. Externally rotate your right leg and draw the right heel up the left inner thigh, until you arrive in tree pose. Just like standing tree pose, move the thigh and foot into each other equally. Can you find balance in the work of all four limbs, even those that are not bearing weight?

Exhale, back to downward-facing dog, and do this vasisthasana tree pose variation again, on the other side.

5. *Malasana Preparation* • Squat
From downward-facing dog, on an exhale jump your feet to the outside of your hands, coming into a malasana preparation. If your heels don't go down, put a small pillow or blanket under them. Deepen the groins and feel the inner knees lifting up.

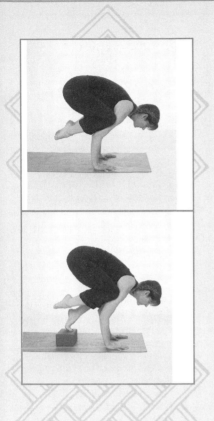

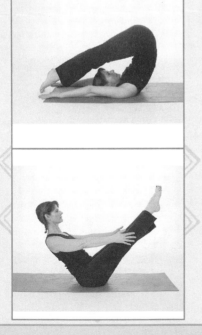

6. *Bakasana* • Crow Pose

For this next pose, think of your hands as your feet. Plant your hands firmly on the floor. Keep your inner thighs on the outside of your upper arms, as high up as you can. Begin to slowly, slowly, slowly, shift your weight forward. Make sure you are looking forward and not dropping your head. Try to lift one foot off the floor. Shift your weight a little bit forward and then try to lift the other foot and bring your toes together. Squeeze your arms with your legs and lift your navel up, rounding your spine slightly.

If you try to jump up into this pose or go too quickly, you will surely fall back down. It is more about feeling the weight shifting and discovering the moment of balance. It is different every day so you have to really pay attention and move mindfully each time. If you are afraid you might fall on your head, place a pillow there, because you might.

A good learning tool for crow pose is a block. Try standing on a block with your feet together. Separate your knees and place your hands on the floor. You may find the pose more accessible this way.

7. *Halasana into Navasana* • Plough Pose into Boat Pose

After you have done crow pose or made a good attempt to do it, let your seat drop to the floor and rock back on your spine into a quick plough pose. Let the momentum rock you up into boat pose. Stay here for five breaths. If your chest is sinking in this position, then bend your knees. Always make the choice that allows your heart and lungs to be supported and most functional.

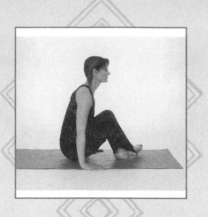

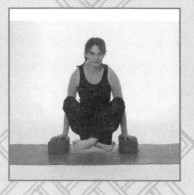

8. *Tolasana Variation* • Lift Up and Jump Back

Exhale and cross your legs. Place your palms on the floor on either side of your hips and on an inhale, lift up off the floor. (If you do this with your legs in lotus, it is full tolasana, which is actually easier for some people.) You might find that you used a lot of effort and still nothing happened—no lifting occurred! Don't worry about it. That's how it starts for many of us. This pose takes a good amount of abdominal strength so you might need to begin by just lifting one foot off the floor.

And I have a good tip for you. Again, it is all about weight distribution. Think architecture and you will realize that you have to swing your pelvis back a bit to balance the weight of the legs in front of you. Try it again. Try placing your hands on blocks to get the feeling of lifting yourself off the floor.

Sit back down, rock forward onto your hands, and as you exhale, jump back to chaturanga. Complete the surya namaskar series.

ADVANCED BALANCING SEQUENCE

As the challenges of this sequence arise, look for balance in your inhalation and exhalation, curiosity and organization.

Stand in tadasana. Inhale and place your hands on your hips. (Sequence is shown with left leg.)

1. *Uttitha Hasta Padangusthasana* • Extended Hand to Foot Pose

Exhale and lift your right thigh up to your chest. Make sure your left leg is still in tadasana and that the left knee is not bending at all. Hold on to your right big toe with the first two fingers of your right hand. This is called yogic toe lock.

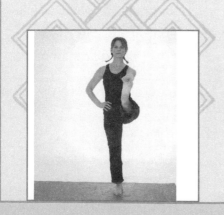

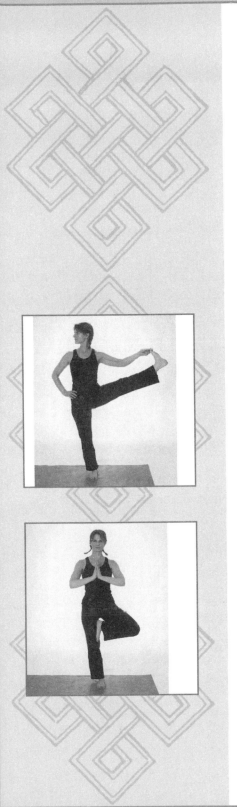

On your next exhale, extend your right leg. Reach out through the foot and at the same time, plug your right thigh bone into the hip socket, finding balance of inward- and outward-moving energies. Don't get confused and think that you will be a happier person if you can get your leg up very high. This is a common misunderstanding. If your spine and standing leg are schlumping in an effort to touch the sky with your right toe tip you will lessen the possibilities for this pose to open for you. You will probably just get stuck in that shape. Can you let go of that? The benefits come from the whole body working in harmony, not one body part dominating.

Open the leg out to the side. Think about trikonasana and how the standing hip tucks under as you externally rotate the right thigh here. Only open the leg as far as you can and still keep both hip points facing forward like headlights.

2. *Vrksasana* • Tree Pose

Release your right hand, bend the right leg, and stand in tree pose. Hook your thumbs and lift the arms up as if they started at the back waist. Try to keep the tongue, throat, and eyes soft.

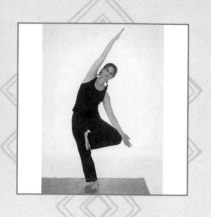

3. Tree Blows in the Wind

Let your right hand float down onto your right thigh and make a small side bend. Feel the movement of this bend. Can you feel your breath more in one side of the ribs than the other?

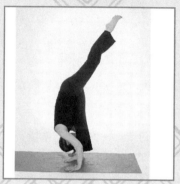

4. *Urdhva Prasarita Ekapadasana* • Standing Split

Inhale back up to vertical and as you exhale, let the leg go up and the torso down at exactly the same time, moving into standing split. The top leg can turn out as much as is possible for you to do and still keep the parallel rotation of the standing leg. If your standing knee had an eye on it you would want to make sure that eyeball was looking straight ahead, not looking to the left or right.

Try balancing here by first holding your left ankle with one hand and then with both. Or try to place your hands on your waist, behind your head or interlaced behind your back. Can you have fun with all that wavering?

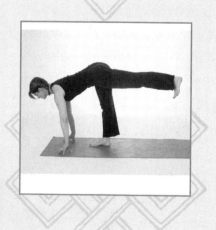

5. *Virabhadrasana 3 Variation* • Warrior 3 Variation

Place both hands on the floor, fingertips in line with toe tips, and rotate the top leg into a warrior 3 alignment, both hip points facing the floor. If you feel strong, try extending your arms alongside your ears and balance in warrior 3 for a breath or two. Try not to harden the breath, even though, at this point, this pose might feel tough.

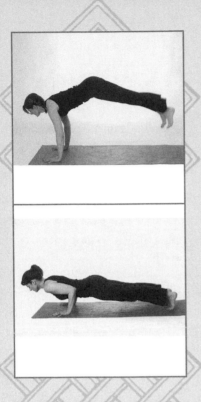

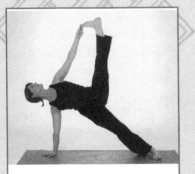

Inhale and bend the front leg. Exhale and jump into chaturanga from here.

Inhale urdhva mukha svanasana (upward-facing dog). (Pictured on page 103.)

Exhale adho mukha svanasana (downward-facing dog). (Pictured on page 104.)

Beginning with #1, repeat sequence on other side up to this point.

6. *Full Vasisthasana* • Full Side Inclined Plane
Shift onto your right hand and the outside of your right foot, again reorganizing the placement of your pelvis so it is in line with your feet and shoulders, just like tadasana. Externally rotate the right leg, bend your knee and take hold of the right foot in yogic toe lock. Extend the right foot up. You will notice that your foot will need to go in front of you somewhat rather than directly up. The angle of the top leg will depend on the amount of external rotation available to you in that hip. This is basically the same pose as uttitha hasta padangusthasana to the side or triangle pose. Roll the upper outer hip crease down and lift the bottom inner thigh. Work toward lifting your hips up high enough to get the bottom foot flat on the floor.

Come back to downward-facing dog. Try this full vasisthasana to the other side and finish in downward-facing dog.

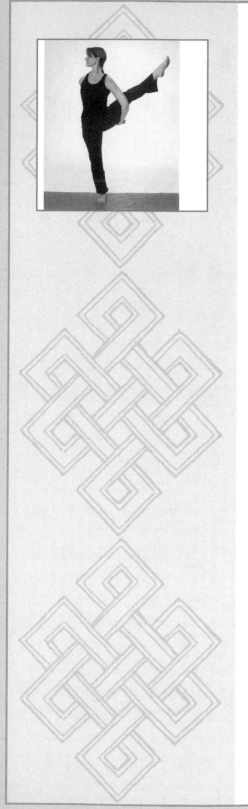

7. *Malasana Variation* • Bird of Paradise

Jump into malasana preparation again. This time lift your hips slightly. Internally rotate your right arm and slip it under your right thigh. Internally rotate your left arm and reach it all the way around behind your back. Try to hold your left wrist with your right hand. Pour your weight into your left foot and, on an inhale, stand up, bringing the right knee up toward the right armpit. Think of dropping your tailbone as you lift your chest and let the balance of this oppositional energy bring you upright. Seeing something at eye level will help you balance.

If you can maintain the foundation of tadasana within this pose, then you can try extending your right leg out to the side and turning your head to the left. Can you manifest the name of this pose? Let your choices be appropriate to what is really available to you today. This is how you begin to develop openheartedness toward yourself as well as honesty and maturity.

Rewind back down to the squat and then try the other side.

From the squat, place your palms on the floor. Exhale, jump into chaturanga.

Move through the advanced sun salute, ending back in tadasana.

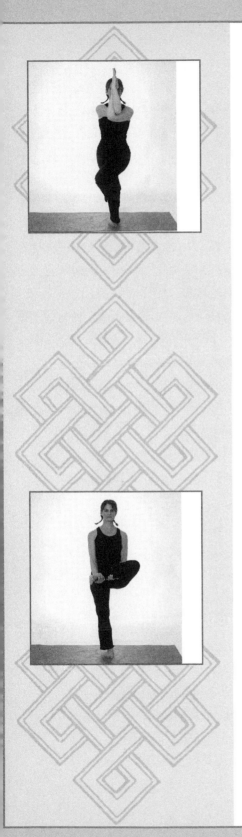

8. *Garudasana* • Eagle Pose

Bend your left leg slightly and lift your right leg up toward your chest. Wrap your right leg around your left leg two times. If you can't do two wraps, do one. You can even work with this pose by keeping the right toe touching the floor. Be mindful that the bottom knee is tracking forward. The arms wrap the opposite way, right arm under left. If your palms cannot face each other but end up in a knot, then place the backs of the hands against each other instead. Eventually your shoulders and wrists will open up.

Soften your gaze and ride the movement of this very wibbly-wobbly pose. Even though the name of this pose is often translated as eagle, in Tibet there is a mythological creature named Garuda. The Garuda is a flying being that never lands. It never lands because it never gets tired. It never gets tired because it rides the wind. Can you ride the wind of your own breath? The quality of the Garuda is that of outrageousness!

9. Standing Pigeon

Release the arms and unwind your right leg. If you are tired, stand down on that leg for a moment, but if not, you can try to keep it lifted. Change the rotation of that thigh from internal to external and hold on underneath your shin. Again, check in to make sure that your tadasana alignment is alive.

After a few breaths, slip your right ankle down so it is just above your left knee. Rest your forearms on your right shin. You are basically standing in utkatasana with the right leg in a hip opening variation. If this is too intense on your right hip, place blocks under your hands. This is how you start to develop the next pose.

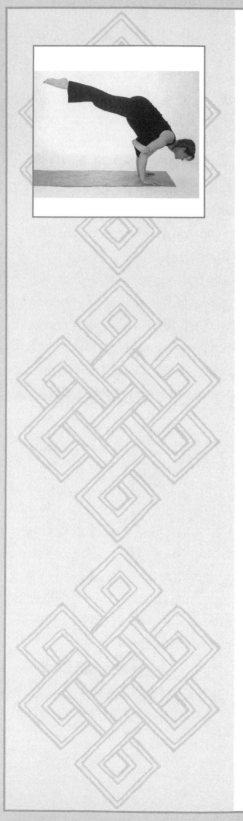

10. *Eka Pada Galavasana* • Flying Crow

Continue to slide your upper arms down the front of your right shin. Hook your right foot around the back of your left upper arm. Fall forward onto your hands, palms flat on the floor. Slowly, just as in crow pose, begin to shift your weight forward so it is completely on your hands. Your back foot will lift up. Keep the knee bent and try to lift your left thigh off your right leg. Then extend the left leg long and up behind you. Sometimes when people are just learning this pose they feel very heavy. Remember that this is a flying pose so try not to get discouraged or too heavy in your efforts. Even if only your breath feels light or your heart or your intention, that's a start.

To release out of this pose, you can just sit down, or step back into downward-facing dog. Over time you might be able to release the front leg and jump back into chaturanga. Repeat steps 8–10 to the other side.

Finish in child's pose.

EIGHT

THE GROUND OF NON-HARMING

Seated Poses

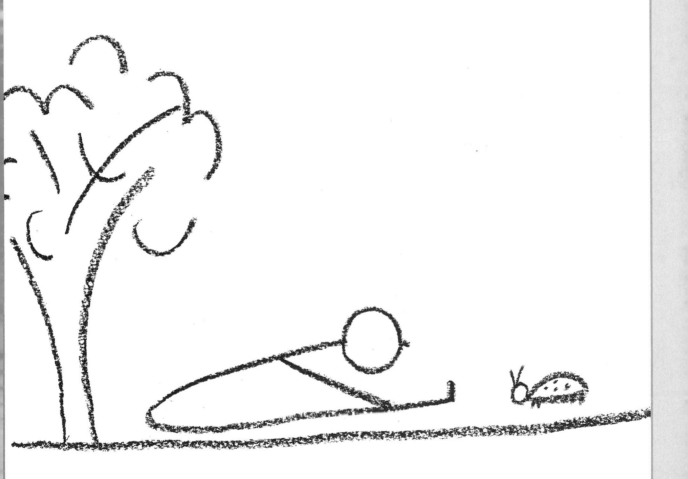

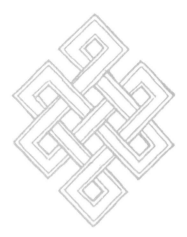

AHIMSA

In yoga practice, we work with oppositional forces. We radiate out and fall back to center, as in warrior 2, we let go to find connection, as in backbends, and we drop down to lift up, as in tree pose. We join heaven—mind, space, vision—with earth—practicality, exertion, manifestation. And we begin that relationship by connecting to the earth in a very real and tangible way. We start with the ground of who and where we are right now. This is a challenge to many of us who don't feel happy with the tightness in our hamstrings, or the weakness in our abdominals. We wish our bodies were different, we wish we were different, and we look to yoga as a self-improvement program.

Yoga and meditation invite us to see who we are right now. The very first step on the path of yoga is found in the yamas and niyamas, the ethical "do's" and "don'ts" set out by Patanjali in his Yoga Sutra. It is ahimsa, which means non-harming to self or others. The first step is also referred to as the ground of the practice, or the foundation from which all other choices evolve. When you commit to practicing ahimsa, you flip the habitual approach to your entire situation, including your attitude toward your own body.

In *The Wisdom of No Escape: And the Path of Loving-Kindness,* Pema Chödron writes, "Practice isn't about trying to throw ourselves away and become something better. It's about befriending who we are already. The ground of practice is you or me or whoever we are right now, just as we are." This is the meaning of ahimsa. It is an invitation to examine our existing condition and let that be the starting place, the finger pointing us in the direction of freedom.

Your back tightness, your squishy tummy, and the irritation and discomfort that arise from your wishing they were different is known as dukha, or suffering. The only way to reverse the claustrophobia of dukha is to acknowledge it. Think about plumbing. Just as the pipes in your house get backed up, creating a flood in your kitchen sink, the pipes of your body need to be kept clean and open. Without unobstructed energy flow we begin to experience tight and tired muscles, slow metabolism, cloudy thinking, and shallow breathing. But you can't repair a clogged drainpipe if you just ignore the stinky sink, or get frustrated and start yelling at it or at whoever is closest to it. You have to take a careful look, see what the problem is, buy the correct tools, and skillfully apply them so the situation is whole and functioning once again.

It's the same with our bodies. If you pretend your legs are loose when they are tight, you will end up straining a back muscle. Your legs will not open more, they will tighten up more. Your pain will increase until the point where you cannot ignore it anymore. This is not ahimsa.

You can begin to reverse that pattern by letting your mindfulness practice and your physical sensations help you understand your body. Then, instead of wishing it were different, let that nonjudgmental information direct you toward appropriate pipe-opening activity, such as pranayama and use of props to enable more movement. Taking a naked look at one's own body and mind, no matter what you find, is the only way to transform dukha, suffering, into sukha, freedom from suffering. Sukha is also translated as space and space is never aggressive or violent.

Letting ahimsa be your guide means, at the very least, don't be a nuisance. We don't often think of ourselves as nuisances to ourselves, but if we take a closer look we might see how we get in the way of our own happiness, how we create our own suffering, through habitual pulling and pushing. This tendency to engage in personal tugs-of-war shows up frequently in seated poses, especially forward bends and hip openers.

BUDDHA MIND

OBSTACLE AS PATH

When I first opened OM Yoga Center I tried to convince students to use props—cushions, blocks, belts, blankets—whatever I felt would be helpful for them and allow them to have the most beneficial experience of their asana practice. OM was one of the few yoga studios in town that incorporated props into a vinyasa form and because this was so new to many of the vinyasa practitioners, there was quite a bit of resistance. Students would rather strain and grunt in an effort to touch their toes, or risk blowing out their back muscles, before they would use a yoga belt, or elevate their pelvis with a block or cushion. They just ignored me when I tried to show them how to create ease in their practice. They thought ease meant easy and that was wimpy. Not enough challenge, boring, too slow.

Over time this pattern began to change through the recognition of dukha, the discomfort that infuses any experience where we ignore the reality of the situation. The way we choose to relate to our bodies can teach us a lot about all of our relationships. In any unhappy relationship, we often feel that we have only two options—endure the pain or drop out of the situation altogether. Using props was a way to practice ahimsa, not causing harm to ourselves or being a nuisance to ourselves with that big lug we call our will. Yoga practice becomes a way to cultivate the understanding that every situation is workable, there are always options. When we recognize that the fight we are engaged in is only a fight with ourselves, then we understand we can take responsibility for creating our own happiness. This understanding will lead to a sense of confidence and freedom that can never be taken from us.

Who can say which comes first, open hips or an open mind? I began to observe that those students who needed props and used them had an opening in their mental approach to the practice. Was it the creation of space in their groins, the relief of strain in the lumbar area, the loosening in their hamstrings that led to the commitment to process over position, or was it the curiosity about what might happen if they tried something different, the willingness to be open to new possibilities? Either way, their relationship to their body, to the goal of their practice, and to their expectations of the yoga experience shifted. The ground of ahimsa—getting out of their own way—led to the fruition of patience, spaciousness, honesty, and maturity. In current lingo, this is called being grounded.

As they learned to place blankets under their sitting bones to create space in the groins, to place blocks under the thighs to prevent knee and groin injuries, to wrap belts around their feet so they could engage their legs and maintain length in their spine, these students had physical openings that led to an opening in their minds about what was right and wrong, desirable or not desirable. It became clear to them that there was a third option to their inner battle of winning or losing, giving up or painfully enduring. The quality of aggressive craving shifted toward a grounded sense of watching the slow, steady opening that happens to everyone who applies ahimsa. What was once viewed as an obstacle—tight hamstrings, rock-hard lower back, locked-up hips—was no longer a problem but a plan. A good, strong, earthy place to start. This can only happen if you shift your goal.

Instead of trying to get rid of obstacles, what if your goal was to work with obstacles creatively? Many people have an idea that meditation is an unchanging state of cottony rapture. Likewise, there is a notion that yoga should be a one-dimensional experience of delicious fluidity and complete physical freedom. This goal-oriented approach sets up a situation where almost everything is an obstacle. But what if your goal is to acknowledge your obstacles and let their nature—the quality, texture, shape—be what wakes you up in that very moment? Then anything that appears to be an obstacle immediately transforms into your path, your direction, your friend. Self-improvement bows to the more interesting self-knowledge. The third option to winning or losing is expanding your options of what makes you happy.

A friend and I were in a café having lunch when suddenly he began choking. I was beginning to be concerned when finally the waiter brought him some water, which he drank, and the choking passed. The waiter asked, "Is that better?" My friend surprised everyone by shaking his head no and simply saying, "It's different." How radical to let the vividness of every single experience be valid, to be open to the flavor of each passing moment, whether bitter or sweet. By staying connected to what is real and tangible, we have even more potential to connect to the space and vision in our heart/mind. Our practice might not be the high of endless rapture and flowing body but we can still get high, an earthy high that is infinite with richness.

Yoga Body

LOCO-(E)MOTION

If the heart center is where we radiate from emotionally, our hips are the heat center from which we radiate out motionally. Yoga anatomy locates the center of our activity prana in our genitals and the element of fire in our pelvis. This heat combined with action extends out through our legs, which become the locomotives that propel us through our world. The ability to generate and sustain movement in this area is one of the main job descriptions of our lower body.

I worked in a physical therapist's office one year and I was surprised to learn that the number one problem bringing people through the door had nothing to do with accidents involving speed, twisting, jumping, or crashing. The main complaint emanated from the opposite situation, lower back pain caused by lack of movement. Day in and day out, the therapists gave back rubs and applied hot packs to loads of people who were perfectly healthy, but their backs were killing them! They all worked at jobs that required them to sit for hours in ill-fitting desk chairs. The therapists would prescribe simple exercises to benefit the body parts related to sitting: lower back, pelvis, hips, and thighs, but most people weren't disciplined enough to do them regularly after the six-week sessions ended.

I suspect that, the rest of the time, those folks never moved anything below the waist except to climb the occasional stair, sit down, stand up, and walk on our hard city sidewalks. We saw return patients over and over again. They had not understood that it wasn't getting out of work to attend their twice-weekly physical therapy that would make the difference. They needed to move.

Our pelvis is home to a lot of movement: digestion, elimination, reproduction. Add on walking, sitting, and breathing and you get the ordinary activities that keep us involved and circulating in our world. Restrict those activities and your entire existence shrinks.

There are lots of reasons—societal and personal—that each of us has for minimizing our pelvic and hip movement. Although the first dictionary definition of hip is the projecting part of each side of the body formed by the pelvis and the upper femur and the flesh covering them, for our purposes we will include genitals, abdomen, lower back, and thighs. Who doesn't have some issue with at least one of those places?

Everywhere we look, advertisements, TV, and film tell us that there is only one good body shape for women and one good body shape for men. No wonder this area is so full of emotional baggage for us. My yoga teacher friend told me her mother lives in her right hip and her father is in her left. Almost everybody wants to change what's going on there—as if that would make us happier. At my gym workouts I see all different kinds of people trying to change their shapes. The thin ones want to get bigger and the soft ones want to get harder. It seems we all want our hips to be smaller or bigger or looser. We want our butts to be firmer or rounder, our bellies to be harder, and our thighs to be dimple-free toothpicks.

We try to change our size and shape without taking the time to really see ourselves as we are and to understand the feelings we have about this area of ourselves.

But as yogis and meditators we can take the approach of ahimsa, beginning that process by increasing our awareness of the current range of motion in our hips, pelvis, lower back, and belly. Start to notice your walking patterns: Do you take long steps or small steps? Do your legs swing freely or does it feel more like your hips are fused to your pelvis as you move? Do you wear tight pants or loose pants? Do you even wear pants? Do you wear tight belts? What kind of shoes do you wear? When was the last time you sat on the floor?

Maybe we can benefit from the advice the Buddha gave the musician by asking him how he tuned his instrument. The reply was, "Not too tight, not too loose." Try reversing your tendency and see how that affects your mobility and attitude about your lower body. If you wear tight pants, go loose for a week, and vice versa. Too loose might mean you're hiding a part of you that you don't like. Try wearing hip huggers for a week, even if only when you're alone at home. Too tight might be cutting off circulation of blood and breath in the lower body. Changing your clothes can begin to change your relationship to your body.

I like the rest of the dictionary definitions for hip: ripe fruit of a wild rose, bramble, or briar; a cheer; and my favorite—being familiar with the latest ideas. The common thread here is an outgoing activity—blossoming, shouting, circulating, and being involved. Just as our upper body is the center for communication, our lower body is our center for locomotion. It contains our ability to manifest the expression of our heart through the world.

Fashion may dictate that we all look the same, but yoga and meditation invite us to be our most authentic, genuine, unique personal self. When we go to a garden, we don't consider only two of the flowers to be beautiful and expect all the others to look like those two. To find our personal balance of earth and heaven, heat and heart, is a individual journey that requires ahimsa, befriending our own being, inside and out.

PRANAYAMA AND THE DANCE OF THE PELVIC FLOOR

"Imagine that you are sitting naked on the ground, with your bare bottom touching the earth. Since you are not wearing a scarf or hat, you are also exposed to heaven above. You are sandwiched between heaven and earth: a naked man or woman, sitting between heaven and earth.

"Earth is always earth. The earth will let anyone sit on it, and the earth never gives way. It never lets you go—you don't drop off this earth and go flying through outer space. Likewise, sky is always sky; heaven is always heaven above you. Whether it is snowing or raining or the sun is shining, whether it is daytime or nighttime, the sky is always there. In that sense, we know that heaven and earth are trustworthy."

These words from Chögyam Trungpa remind us that the earth holds us all without discrimination. She is truly Mother Earth. When that understanding sinks in, we can also sink in; into the soft support of the mother earth. When we walk or sit or stand or lie down on the earth, we can always trust this to be true and so we can begin to relax a little bit.

You may notice, especially if you live in an urban or suburban environment where you walk on concrete surfaces, that your abdominal muscles are constantly contracting in an unconscious effort to protect your organs from being jostled. Our bodies are in a sort of physical holding pattern of forced uplift because there is no organic rebound from the earth's energy. We grip to try to stay up because cement does not support us and we can feel intuitively that if we drop down into it, we will tend to collapse down and stay there. That is not relaxing, but going unconscious.

To avoid this we apply the holding-up mode, which causes our breath to remain shallow. It's like inhaling without exhaling and in fact, many of us do not ever exhale completely. In order to let the breath flow freely and to find balance, through inhale and exhale, down and up, earth and heaven, we need to create the conditions for breathing to happen by yielding to the earth.

Sir Isaac Newton said, "To every action there is an equal and opposite reaction." Relaxing into the safety of the earth will create the conditions for breathing to happen. In fact, one of the synonyms for relax in the thesaurus is "breathe easy." The natural fall will lead to a natural rise and this rhythm will infuse each step, each breath, each heartbeat.

The element of fire in our pelvic belly relates to creative passion as well as more earthy things like the digestive process. If there is no movement in this area it gets tight, inhibiting the flow of the breath. Without the air element of the breath the digestive fire cannot ignite leading to problems such as constipation, lower back pain, sciatica, or even more serious issues.

Pranayama, the yogic art of breathing, is defined by yoga master B. K. S. Iyengar like this: "Prana means energy and ayama means the storing or distributing of the energy." Prana is vital energy in the universe that is received by us through sunlight, water, food, earth. One of the easiest ways for us to consciously access prana is through breathing exercises. The two main directions of our internal air circulation are prana, the upward-moving wind, and apana, the downward-moving wind. Prana happens on the inhalation and relates to the upper body and has the qualities of nourishing and building. Apana, exhalation, moves away from the brain and relates to the activities of eliminating and removing.

Balance is achieved when the prana, inhaling, and the apana, exhaling, are in balance. The following pranayama exercise will help you to experience these movements in your body, particularly in the muladhara chakra, located at the base of the spine, which is the source and support of vital force, and the svadisthana chakra, located at the genital organs, the seat of vital force.

Lie down on your back with your knees bent, feet flat on the floor. Extend your arms up alongside your head, palms facing up. Lengthen your waist as much as possible, making space between your ribs and your pelvis. Let your shoulder blades move into your rib cage, softly opening the chest.

Now circle your arms down by your sides and place your fingertips on your lower belly, about two inches above your pubic bone. Feel the movement of your breath through the waters of your pelvis. As you exhale, pay attention to the tailbone and feel how it curls up slightly and tones the pelvic floor. Can you feel how your pelvic floor is a diaphragm that moves up and down just like the diaphragm between your visceral organs and your heart and lungs? Imagine your exhalation being initiated at the pelvic floor. Continue breathing like this for at least a couple of minutes.

Now bring your knees up toward your armpits. You will find that your back arches slightly and this is fine. There should be enough space between your lower back and the floor for a friendly mouse to run through. This position allows the pubic bone to reach through the thighs toward the ground, which in turn hollows the groins and allows for a deeper inhalation. Can you feel the in-breath dropping the pubic bone and then filling up the torso and lifting the heart? Continue to explore this breath for a few minutes.

Eventually see if you can feel the lift of the tailbone—the action of the exhale—during the inhale. Try to be sensitive enough to feel the dropping of the pubic bone and the lift of the heart even as the exhale tucks the tail slightly. In other words, just as in asana we drop down to extend up, in pranayama we look for the inhalation within the exhalation, and observe how the exhalation informs the inhalation.

This subtle pulsing of firmness and fluidity creates a dance of breath which tones the muscles of the pelvic floor. The more breath and consciousness we can awaken in this area, the more confidence we will have as we begin to really snuggle down into the earth with true awakened relaxation.

You can practice this anywhere anytime, waiting for the bus, sitting on the bus, driving the bus. Explore the movement of your pelvis within the privacy of your own pants. Get to know your movement and breath limitations and watch how they change depending on the situation, outfit, and awareness. Look for expression from all the elements of life—the earth of our bony sacroiliac, the watery ocean of our organs, the flowing air of apana, the heat of our digestive fire.

Here's an earthy (in other words, practical) tip for creating opening in the pelvis, hips, and lower back: Get off your chair and sit on the floor as much as possible. I have one student who took this advice to heart. He got rid of his office chair and now works sitting cross-legged *on* his desk, instead of at his desk. He and his hips have opened up a lot. That's a perfect example of starting where you are.

In no way does it matter if your hips are tight or loose. Start your hip opening practice by being kind to yourself. Then be honest and allow the situation at hand to dictate whether you need props in order to create the conditions for opening in your pelvis and deepening in your breathing. Rest with where you are. Feel the unconditional support of the earth. Watch how things open naturally when you give them support, attention, time, and prana.

Maybe, like my student, you will also find that letting ahimsa be your foundation will create the space that leads to creative solutions. This is the first step on the path to transforming obstacles into a new way of moving through the world. This is the ground of our practice.

SEATED POSES, HIP OPENERS, AND TWISTS

Let the part of you that's called "your seat," the part you actually sit on, connect to the earth. Notice if your hip points are lifted, if there is breath in your pelvic belly, if there is mobility in your hip joints. If not, then your starting place is telling you to use props.

Here's how to use props for seated poses:

- Blanket or block: The guidelines of tadasana still apply even though we are now sitting down. Look for a balanced relationship between your pubic bone and tailbone. If you are tucked under, your back muscles will have to work too hard to keep your spine vertical. Place your sitting bones so that your spine can easily grow up out of your pelvic bowl.

  Anytime your hips are not balanced (such as in bharadvajasana and pigeon, both coming up) and you feel like you are tipping over, place a firm and neatly folded blanket or cushion under the levitating hip. Let the blanket be the earth rising up to meet you and hold you. Now you can relax your weight down into the blanket or cushion which will make the corresponding upward support of the earth be available to you. If one cushion is not enough you can also try sitting on a block.

- Belt: If you cannot reach your feet in seated forward bends, then use a belt, long tie, or towel. Again, you want to maintain the length of your spine, openness of your heart and lungs, and activity of the legs and arms, just as if you were in tadasana. If you let go of this work due to striving for a goal such as touching your toes, you will lessen your ability to receive the full benefits of the pose.

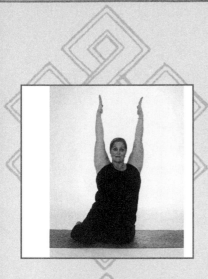

BEGINNER SEATED SEQUENCE

1. *Bharadvajrasana* • Bharadvajra's Pose
Inhale, arms up next to your ears.

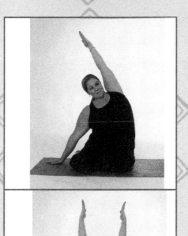

2. *Bharadvajrasana with Side Bend Variation*
Exhale, bend to the right. Take your left arm over your ear but keep your left hip connected to the ground. If you feel as though you might tip over, place a cushion under your lifted hip.

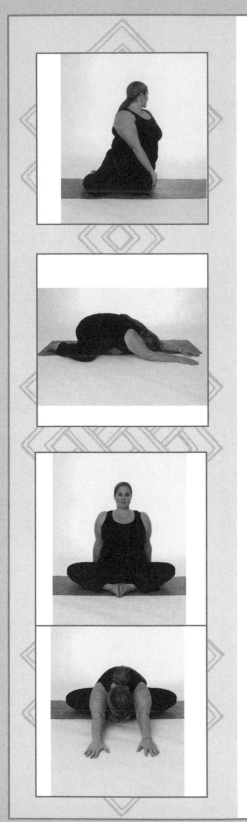

3. *Bharadvajrasana Twist*

Inhale, arms and body back up to vertical.

Exhale, twist to the left.

4. Hip Opener/Forward Bend

Inhale, arms up facing forward.

Exhale, open one knee and fold forward.

5. *Baddhakonasana* • Bound Angle or Cobbler's Pose

Inhale, sitting back up, letting your arms stay down. Lift your top leg and turn it out, bringing the soles of your feet together. This can happen all in that same big inhale.

Exhale, walk your hands forward and fold over.

Inhale, use your hands to walk yourself back up to sitting.

Stay for three to five breaths in each of the following asanas:

(1–5 can be repeated as warm-up vinyasa.)

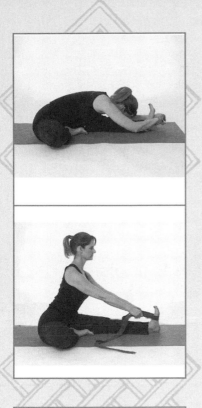

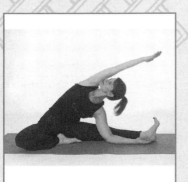

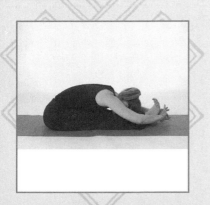

6. *Janu Sirsasana* • Head to Knee Pose

From baddhakonasana, straighten your left leg out in front of you. Inhale as you lift and lengthen your spine. Fold over on an exhale. Even though this is called "head to knee," think of reaching the top of your head toward your foot, so your chest doesn't get closed in.

Hold on to your shin, ankle, foot—wherever you can reach without rounding your back or bending your knee. This may require that you loop a belt around your foot. You may also need to sit on a blanket. Remember these yoga *accessories* make the pose *accessible* and allow you to *access* its wonderful benefits.

7. *Parivirtta Janu Sirsasana* • Rotated Head to Knee Pose

Still folded over, you can now dip your left shoulder down in front of your left knee, or something near there that you can reach. Inhale, lift your right arm up and over your top ear. Each time you exhale, you may find that you can spin your belly a little bit more up toward the ceiling.

8. *Pascimottanasana* • Intense West Stretch

This asana stretches the entire back of your body, which in yoga is called the west. The back of your body includes the soles of your feet, the back of your legs, the back of your torso, neck, and your head all the way up and around to the space between your eyes. Inhale to lift the spine, and exhale to fold forward, again using whatever props may be helpful

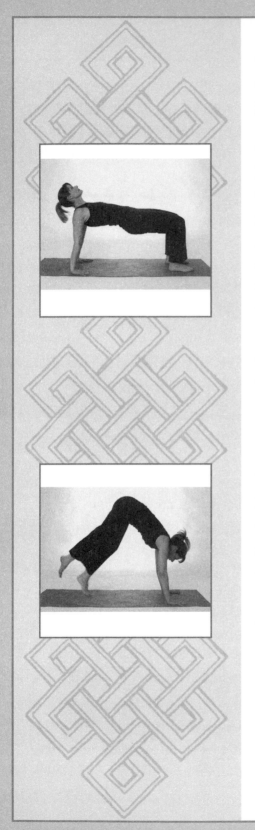

to you today. If you feel strain in any of those areas, pull back on your effort. Discriminate between strain, sensation, grasping, opening. Watch, wait, and breathe.

9. *Purvottanasana Variation* • Intense East Stretch

Place your palms about eight inches behind you. Press down with your hands and feet as you inhale to lift up. Keep looking forward and check that your knees are tracking directly forward. Instead of gripping your buttocks, which is an unconscious impulse, press down with your feet even more, trying to activate the back of your legs. Imagine breathing through your sacrum.

Sit back down on an exhale and swing your legs to the left to begin this entire sequence (1–9) on the other side.

INTERMEDIATE SEATED SEQUENCE

Begin with surya namaskar through the first downward-facing dog.

From downward-facing dog jump into seated spinal twist like this: Jump forward onto your right foot. Tuck your left knee down on the outside of your right foot and have a seat. Practice so that eventually you can do it all in one movement.

Remain in each of the following poses for three to eight breaths.

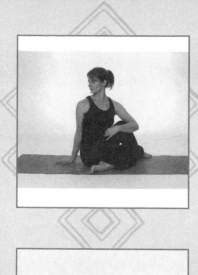

1. *Matsyendrasana* • Lord of the Fishes or Seated Spinal Twist
Make sure both sitting bones are connected to the earth. Use a blanket if you can't get them both down. In the twist, try to feel equal length and breath in both sides of the ribs. Be mindful that the wrapping around arm doesn't pull that hip up off the floor. Soften your neck, throat, and eyes. Stay here for 3–5 breaths.

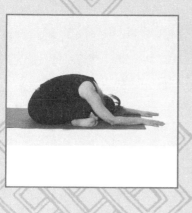

2. Ankle to Knee Pose
The ankles and knees align with each other, right knee over left ankle, and left knee all the way forward directly below your right ankle. Flex your feet actively as if you were standing on the four corners of your feet.

This pose is a challenge for most of us. This might be a good time to sit on a block. The sensations of this pose can sometimes be so intense that you might find yourself tightening or holding in ways that are not necessary. Scan your body and let go where you can. 3–5 breaths.

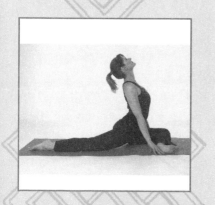

3. *Eka Pada Raja Kapotasana* • One-Legged Pigeon
Swing the top leg in ankle to knee pose all the way around behind you to bring you into pigeon pose. Check for these alignment points: back leg extending directly back, not out to the side; top of the foot on the floor, not rolling in or out; both hip points and nipples pointing forward. If you have organized your pose this way and now find that your bent leg hip is hovering off the floor, you know what to do—slip a block or cushion underneath it.

Walk your hands back beside your hips, inhale to lift the

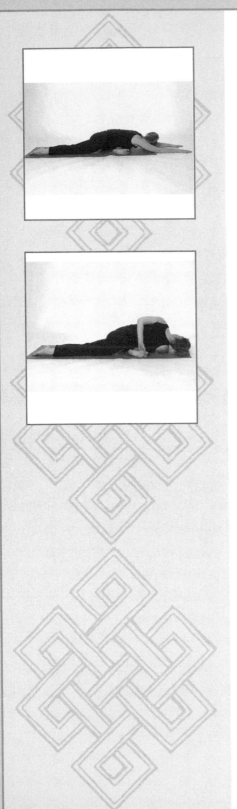

spine, and exhale, rippling through every single vertebra as you walk your hands forward and fold over. 5 breaths.

4. Eka Pada Raja Kapotasana with a Twist

After a few breaths in pigeon, walk your hands in a bit, slip your right arm under your left armpit, and place your right shoulder on the floor. Your left palm can cover your right; keeping your fingertips touching, exhale into a twist. The twist will begin at the low spine and move up until you begin to draw that top shoulder back, straightening the left arm.

For fun, you can then extend your left arm up to the ceiling, internally rotating it. Reach behind your back and see if you can take hold of the left big toe.

Untwist, place your palms under your shoulders, and inhale back up.

5. Janu Sirsasana • Head to Knee Pose

Swing your back leg around in front of you. Place your left foot either against your upper right thigh (can you see the relationship between this pose and tree pose?), or you can open your left thigh out into a 100-degree angle, with your left heel in your left groin. Maintain activity in your right leg as if it were in tadasana. Align your spine over your straight leg as much as possible and you will notice that this is a mild twist. Exhale, and fold over your straight leg. (Pictured on page 154.)

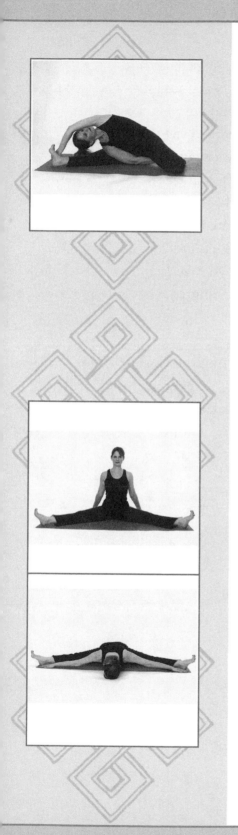

6. *Virasana Parivritta Janu Sirsasana* • Rotated Head to Knee Pose with Half Hero Leg

Inhale, up from janu sirsasana. Use your hands to help you lift your hips up. Slide your pelvis forward, rolling over your bent leg, and sitting back down in half virasana. Separate your thighs as much as possible. Place your hands on the floor in front of you and again lift your hips. Slip your right arm under your pelvis and take hold of your left ankle. Dip your right shoulder down in front of your right knee, spin your belly to the left, and extend your left arm up as you lower your seat back down.

If this pose is not available to you right now, you can try it sitting up on a block, or you can do parivritta janu sirsasana, as in the beginner sequence. (Pictured on page 155.)

7. *Upavista Konasana* • Seated Open Angle

Inhale and sit up. Release your bottom hand. Keep your left heel close to your left hip as you lift your left knee and bring the thigh back around in the original janu sirsasana position. From here extend your left leg out and open to the side.

Sit up tall—use an accessory, if necessary. Slowly begin to walk your hands forward. Be mindful that your legs are active, and that your knees and toes are pointing up, not rolling forward or back. As you slide your pubic bone back, keep the sitting bones and buttock flesh dropping earthward. Watch your breath and see how slowly but surely your body moves and opens.

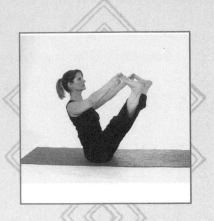

8. *Upavista Navasana* • Open Angle Boat Pose

Take hold of your big toes in yogic toe lock—first two fingers of each hand wrapped around your big toes. Inhale and lift right up with straight legs into open angle boat pose. This is a full-body coordination—reach out through your feet as you pull your shoulders back; lift your chest as you rock back on your sitting bones. Give it five tries and then if you can't do it, bend your legs to come into this pose. Over time you will get it, but don't frustrate yourself today.

Strongly reach through your heels and come back down into upavista konasana, landing on your calves, not your heels. Inhale, and sit back up.

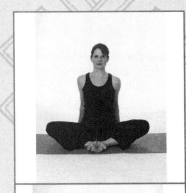

9. *Baddhakonasana* • Bound Angle or Cobbler's Pose

Place your hands inside your knees and lift them up to bring your feet together for baddhakonasana. Try to deepen the envelope of inner knee bend as you press the outer edges, or baby toe sides, of your feet together.

Exhale, and slowly, attentively, fold forward. No aggression, please.

Inhale to come back up.

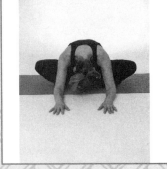

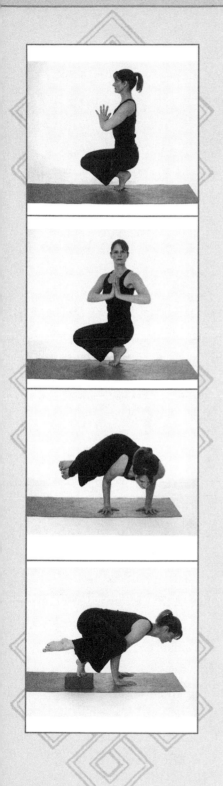

10. *Parsva Bhakasana* • Side Crow Pose

Bring your knees and the inner edges of your feet together. Lift your spine so that you are vertical in a little chair position. Twist to the left, checking that your knees stay together and pointing forward, as your chest and shoulders face to the right. Place your hands on the floor, right baby finger in line with left baby toe and left hand shoulder distance out to the left. Your hands will need to be about twelve inches away from your feet so you have space to lift your hips up onto your right arm. Your left arm is there for balance but does not support your hips at all.

If you are having trouble getting up on your arm, try standing on a block to do this. This way your hips are already on the level of your upper arm and you can start to get the feeling for how to do this pose.

This is a combo of bharadvajasana with chaturanga arms. Now you are no longer sitting on the ground but you still need to connect to the earth in the same way by reaching down with your palms. This downward reach will help you to feel the lifting up of the arm muscles on the arm bones, the rolling back of the shoulders, the lift of the belly creating a slight spinal curve, and the lightness in the pelvis as you sit on your arm.

Give it a try three times and then relax. If you don't get it today, you can try it again tomorrow.

Step into downward-facing dog and complete surya namaskar, moving through either astang pranam (knees-chest-chin) and baby cobra, or chaturanga and upward-facing dog, before arriving in downward-facing dog. Take three breaths and at the end of the third exhale, jump forward and finish surya namaskar, ending in tadasana, ready to repeat this sequence on the second side.

ADVANCED SEATED SEQUENCE

Begin with surya namaskar through downward-facing dog.

From downward-facing dog, jump through your arms with straight legs, landing in dandasana. Here's how to work on that jump through: In downward-facing dog take a big breath in and near the end of your exhale, bend your knees and begin to jump your feet toward the space between your hands. When your feet get there inhale to shoot the legs through and exhale as you land on your seat in dandasana.

1. *Dandasana*
This is the foundation for all seated poses, just as tadasana is for all standing poses. You can see that they are basically the same pose, only bent at the hips.

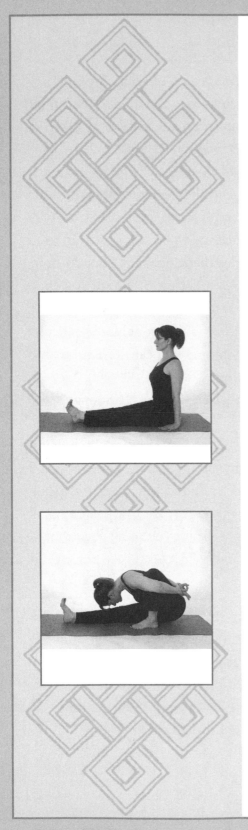

(Sequence is shown on left side.)

2. *Marichyasana 1* • Marichi's Pose 1
Place your right foot on the floor, about a fist distance away from your left thigh, bringing your right heel in line with your right sitting bone. Left leg stays active in dandasana. Inhale, and lengthen your spine. As you exhale, bend forward and extend your right arm forward; internally rotate it, turning the palm away from you. Wrap that arm around the outside of your right leg. As you internally rotate your left arm and reach it behind you, let the left shoulder and armpit chest area open to the left a little bit, too. Try to hold on to your left hand with your right wrist. If you can't reach it, use a belt. Square off your shoulders to the front and exhale as you fold forward.

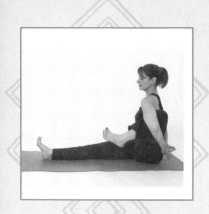

3. Ankle Rotation

Keep your arms in the bound position as you sit up on an inhale. Again, try to stay lifted on your sitting bones, with an open chest. Roll your ankle four times in each direction.

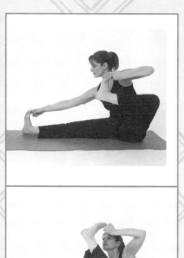

4. *Akarna Dhanurasana* • Bow and Arrow

Release the arm bind and take hold of both toes in yogic toe lock. Exhale, and draw the right leg back, bringing your right toe close to your right ear. Inhale, and extend the right foot straight up. You can stay in each position for a few breaths and repeat this again a couple of times.

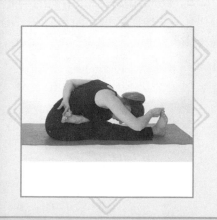

5. *Ardha Padmasana Pascimottanasana* • Half Lotus Forward Bend

Externally rotate the right leg and place it in half lotus. Think of moving the thighs toward each other, almost as if they would become parallel to each other. Wrap your right arm behind you and hold on to your right toe. Again, use a belt if you can't reach.

Hold on to your left leg wherever you can reach while still maintaining integrity in your alignment. If you can do that and hold on to your left toe, then try that. Inhale to prepare, and exhale to fold forward. Inhale to sit up.

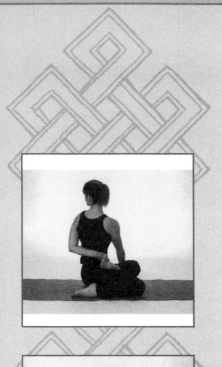

6. *Full Bharadvajrasana Bound Twist*

Bend your left leg behind you. This is the full version of the very first pose we did in the beginning of the seated poses sequences. Twist to the right on the exhale.

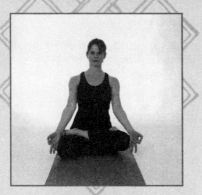

7. *Padmasana* • Full Lotus

Release your arms. Mindfully rotate your bottom leg and bring it around for full lotus. As you work on this pose, take time and care so your knees don't get hurt at all. No pulling or tugging, please. If your hips are tight, you can work on half lotus. Let this be a long-term project.

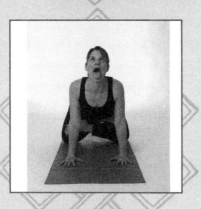

8. *Simhasana 2*

Either in full lotus, half lotus, or easy crossed legs, shift forward onto your hands. Let your tailbone slip toward your pubic bone as you lift your belly slightly and open your chest, a bit like upward-facing dog. Inhale, and as you exhale, stick your tongue out and down toward your chin and roll your eyes up to the space between your eyebrows. Fun!

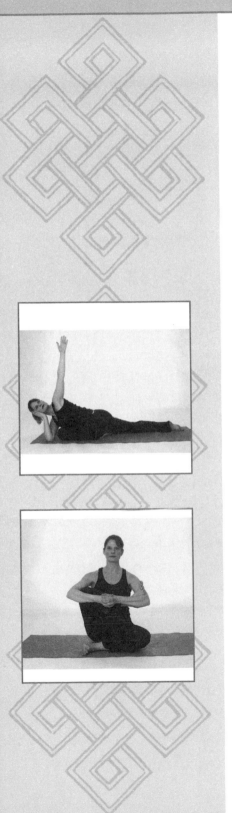

Either rock back and lift up into tolasana (page 131), swing your hips back, and jump into chaturanga; or rock back, cross your legs, then rock forward onto your hands and jump back into chaturanga. Then upward-facing dog and downward-facing dog.

Repeat from the beginning of the sequence, on your second side, before continuing.

Proceed from downward-facing dog:

9. *Eka Pada Raja Kapotasana with Twist* • Pigeon with Twist
Bring your right knee into your chest, externally rotate it, and come into pigeon pose. Keep your spine up and as you exhale, twist toward your front knee. Place your left elbow on the floor and your left cheek in your hand. Spin your left ribs under to increase the twist on your next exhale and float the right arm up to the sky. This development of the pigeon twist in the intermediate class is a huge hip opener!

10. Cradle Leg and Touch Foot
Exhale and untwist. Swing your back leg around and in front of you. Cradle it with your arms, rocking it back and forth like a precious baby. After a few breaths here, hold on to your foot. Bring your toe to (or toward) the space between your eyebrows, your nose, the hollow of your throat, your heart center, your belly button. Make sure you stay sitting tall and don't bring your forehead down to your toe!

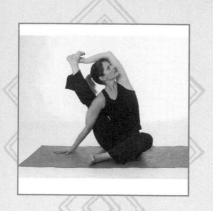

11. *Visvamitrasana Variation* • Compass Pose

Place your right knee on your right shoulder, or as high up on your right arm as you can. Plant your right hand on the floor using the right arm to anchor the thigh in place. Hold on to the outside of your right foot with your left hand. Exhale and extend the right foot straight up. Spin your belly to the left and look up to the left.

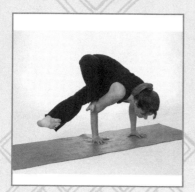

12. Mystery Arm Balance

Release out of compass and place your right ankle on your left thigh. Bend your left leg, shift your weight forward, and come up into a one-legged chair pose. Twist to the left and place your right upper arm in the sole of your right foot. From here lean toward the floor and place your palms on the floor with your arms in a chaturanga configuration—with your right foot still on your right upper arm. Now you are basically standing on your right upper arm. Extend your left leg out. Wow!

Work on this for a while and you will get it soon.

Sit back. Jump back to chaturanga, then move through the vinyasa, transitioning to the other side. Repeat (9–12).

After your last downward-facing dog, lower your knees to the floor and rest in child's pose.

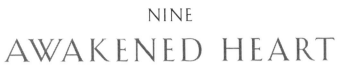

NINE

AWAKENED HEART

Backbending

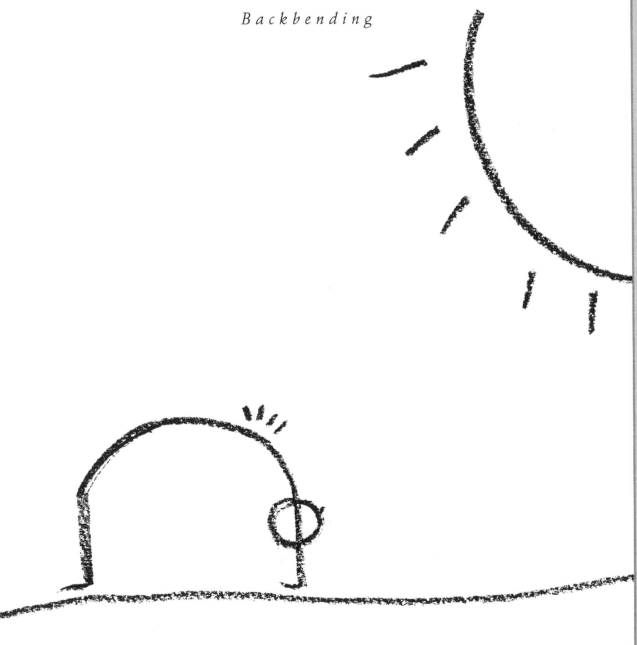

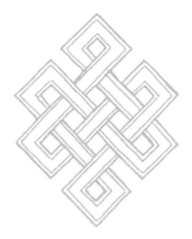

Buddha Mind

MOTION TO EMOTION

The summer before my first marriage broke up I cried a lot in yoga class. When we lay down for the final relaxation, tears would pour out of the sides of my eyes. It was almost like I wasn't crying, but leaking, and it happened every day for the whole summer. Somehow the release of effort in my muscles and toxins in my organs led to the release of emotions in my heart and mind. Motion led to emotion. Before the class I was stuck and yoga unstuck me. It took me on a journey back to myself. As I embodied my sadness more and more, it traveled back out of me and by the end of the summer, I felt clean, balanced, and brave enough to make the necessary changes in my life.

It turned out that even though it was painful, my summer of being heartbroken was better than having no heart at all. I recently introduced my girlfriend, who is a hardcore type A, to yoga. At the end of the class, she told me, "I felt my heart! For the first time in my life, I felt my heart beating inside my chest." This woman has done aerobics for years, jogging, weightlifting, golfing, you name it, but it took the sensitivity and stillness of yoga for her to experience her own heartbeat. This was a powerful moment for her, as it is for all of us when we truly experience the movement of our heart. Even if our heart feels sadness or fear or anger, that is how we know we are alive. When we don't experience this circulation of emotions, we get depressed and then stuck there. My friend had made other more conceptual efforts to connect to herself—psychotherapy, twelve steps—but the physical approach took her right to the immediacy of her own beating heart.

One of my yoga students, a classic New York East Villager with a shaved head, pierced nose, ears, and tongue, and many tattoos, seemed intimidating except that he was so obviously into yoga and eager to learn more. One day in class he timidly asked, "Is the reason that backbending is so difficult for me because my heart is closed?" In that moment, I saw how tender and delicate he was. I almost felt like crying, and could feel that the whole class was moved. That tough exterior was very effective armor for a fragility that had finally gained the courage to expose itself. I said, "No. I don't think you are hard-hearted at all. But your muscles are tight, and we can work with that."

Of all the workshops I offer around the world, the Heart Opener tends to fill up the quickest. I find that quite moving, because I feel sure that the people who sign up for those workshops are already openhearted. It is just that the supporting anatomy may be tight or weak, so it can be difficult to feel the physical movement that enables our emotional journey to deepen.

Try this. Sit up tall and take a deep breath in. As you exhale, schlump—tailbone tucked under, shoulders curving forward—and try to take in another deep breath. No matter how hard you try, you really can't do it, and the effort begins to be disheartening. As your spine droops, your head drops, your spirit sinks. You can't see the sky or meet the world head-on.

The Sanskrit word for heart is *hridayam*, which means "that which receives, gives, and circulates." The anatomical function of the heart does exactly that. It receives deoxygenated blood from the veins, pumps blood into the lungs where it gets oxygenated, and circulates the oxygenated blood to the arteries and on through the entire system.

The functions of the heart and lungs are intimately related through this exchange, and as we learned in our breathing experiment, we cannot inhale enough air when our cardiovascular department is compressed. This inability to take in oxygen is a subtle form of suffocation, and leads to weak prana or life force. Ayurvedic medicine says that our "life prana" resides in our heart.

We often picture our mind in our head and our heart in our chest. But just as our consciousness inhabits our entire being so does our heart. In fact, in Tibetan the word for mind and heart is the same. If your heart is everywhere in your body, then it's really not that difficult to feel it once you become sensitive enough. Close your eyes, rest your mind, and begin to explore how many places in your body you can feel your pulse—temples, neck, chest, abdomen, groins, back of the knees—anywhere else?

We can begin to increase this felt understanding of giving, receiving, and circulating by strengthening the supportive and protective anatomy around our heart and extending the range of motion in those areas. That includes our arms, rib cage, shoulders, neck, upper back, and chest. First we have to notice that we even have those body parts.

Our arms, in particular, are the expression of our heart. They allow us to communicate, gesture, embrace, and protect. A study done by someone somewhere said that only 7 percent of communication occurs through words, and that 93 percent is through our bodies and our hearts. Even though I don't know who did that study, I know it's true. Think waving, pointing, catching, hailing a cab, holding a baby, and our favorite—hugging—because that's when our heart centers touch. Give yourself a hug right now by wrapping one arm over the other. See if you can reach your shoulder blades, then shrug your shoulders and separate the shoulder blades a little bit more. Deepen your breath and send it into the space between your shoulder blades, opening up the back of the heart and the muscles of the upper back.

Our shoulder and neck department relates to the more conceptual part of ourselves—the masculine quality of outward-moving activity—that tends to work too hard and get tired and tense. When this happens, our shoulders tend to climb up our necks and eat our ears. This area is such a popular tension spot that, according to New York mythology, the city's cabdrivers don't even have necks anymore.

Put this book down right now and give yourself a little massage. Place your hands on the top of your back and begin to palpate your trapezius, the muscles at the very top of your back that run from your neck to your shoulders. From there walk your fingers up the back of your neck. Explore this part of your spine, and see if your vertebrae feel balanced. Continue up to the base of the skull, around behind the ears, back down the sides of the neck, and begin to feel your collarbones. Did you know your lungs go all the way up past your collarbones? Can you feel your breath and your heart beat in the front of your neck? What is it like to massage the tender muscles on the front of your neck? Use the opposite hand to give each shoulder and arm a little massage. This is a great way to increase circulation as well as awareness in all of these areas.

Your shoulders, arms, neck, and ribs can be either a restrictive cage for your heart, or an undulating, comforting protector. Well-known yoga teacher Rodney Yee once asked a class, "If you could hold your heart in your hands, how would you hold it?" Ask yourself how you hold it now: tightly, tenderly, firmly and gently, carefully and attentively? Do I grip it or give it space?

OPENING IS SCARY

Last Halloween, one of the teachers at OM Yoga Center began his evening class by inviting students to request yoga poses they found scary. He was not surprised by fancy suggestions such as bending backward to touch the head to the floor; standing on one's arms instead of legs; five-minute headstands; and, of course, various pretzels in the leg-behind-the-neck category. But the entire class was a little surprised when one of the students requested meditation, saying, "That's the scariest part of yoga."

Pema Chödron, in her book *The Places That Scare You,* reminds us that "the Buddha taught that flexibility and openness bring strength and that running from groundlessness weakens us and brings pain." She asks, "But do we understand that becoming familiar with the running away is the key? Openness doesn't come from resisting our fears, but from getting to know them well."

Some of us run away by avoiding our own mind/heart while others like to run away from their external environments. Some of us do both without even knowing it. Once a year you can find me leaving New York City with a dharma book, a yoga mat, and a tension headache, off to lead a yoga retreat in Costa Rica. The open-air studio where I teach there is filled with a sensuous composition of sweet birdsong, ripening fruit, and fragrant flowers. I cross my legs, sit down on the almond tree floor, and feel healthy, inspired, and nurtured from the quiet and the space.

Then I come home to downtown Manhattan where the air quality makes me nauseous and construction work shakes my whole building. I wake up to fire engine sirens roaring out of the station on the next block. I go to sleep listening to drunken hipsters at the snobby restaurant outside my bedroom window. I inhale car fumes from the mechanic's garage downstairs, I shower over the rumbling of the subway. Even though I love New York, it's a challenge to let in this barrage of toxicity. Is it really true that I will feel more openhearted and flexible in both body and mind if I can be brave enough to let in difficulty rather than shutting it out?

Whether the environmental rubs are external or internal, opening is scary because it comes under the category of being rather than doing. We are all used to managing our experience and are generally comfortable with a project mentality. This approach allows us to think that we are controlling our experience, in other words, that things are in control. For many experienced hatha yogis, sitting still in meditation requires more effort, more courage, than doing 108 sun salutations. For others, opening up to traffic, family expectations, or noisy neighbors is the toughest challenge.

The basic premise of yoga is union, and, for most of us, the idea of connecting to everything and everyone sounds inspiring and beautiful, until we encounter irritation. Then we begin to pick and choose who and what we want to consider ourselves related to. Unfortunately, choosing doesn't really work because we end up being pulled like taffy back and forth between our cravings for what attracts us and our rejection of what seems icky or scary. Divine union doesn't mean we should figure out what is divine and just get with that. It means everything is divine—including us—and when we can be brave enough to relax our judgments, our opinions, our fears, we once again feel that divinity, harmony, flow, and strength.

The Buddha's First Noble Truth says that suffering exists, but none of us needs a Buddhist to tell us that. We all know the feeling of disappointment, broken heart, rejection, and loss. Kisagotami's story reminds us that we are not alone in our suffering:

"In the time of the Buddha, a woman named Kisagotami suffered the death of her only child. Unable to accept it, she ran from person to person, seeking a medicine to restore her child to life. The Buddha was said to have such a medicine. Kisagotami went to the Buddha, paid homage, and asked, "Can you make a medicine that will restore my child?"

"I know of such a medicine," the Buddha replied. "But in order to make it, I must have certain ingredients."

Relieved, the woman asked, "What ingredients do you require?"

"Bring me a handful of mustard seed," said the Buddha. The woman promised to secure it for him, but as she was leaving, he added, "I require the mustard seed be taken from a household where no child, spouse, parent, or servant has died."

The woman agreed and began going from house to house in search of the mustard seed. At each house the people agreed to give her the seed, but when she asked them if anyone had died in that household, she could find no home where death had not visited. In one house a daughter, in another a servant, in others a husband or parent had died. Kisagotami was not able to find a home free from the suffering of death. Seeing she was not alone in her grief, the mother let go of her child's lifeless body and returned to the Buddha, who said with great compassion, "You thought that you alone had lost a son. The law of death is that among all living creatures there is no permanence."

Ironically it's our own suffering that is the seed of compassion. His Holiness the Dalai Lama says everyone on earth wants the same thing—to be happy. The path to happiness comes when we can begin to reverse our habitual tendency to do whatever it takes to create our own pleasure and instead try to help others. When we close ourselves off from others either because we have a chemical reaction to them or because they didn't do what we wanted them to exactly how and when we wanted it, our potential for happiness diminishes. The conditions for our happiness become too specific and small. This is how we get stuck and lose the experience of movement, the wordless understanding that grasping will not lead to joy, but only create fear. Our own happiness flows more freely when we take the focus off of ourselves and put it onto others. Once we have begun to feel our own heart, we can begin to remind ourselves, just as Kisagotami did, that others have hearts, too.

The first step toward awakening our heart is to quietly pay attention. But if that is as deep as we go we will only know half of our heart's story. The job of the heart is to circulate: to both give and receive. One of the most amazing things about being a yoga teacher is when I make hands-on adjustments on students, I sometimes feel their heart beating. It is so tiny and strong at the same time. I am moved that that little pulsation is what keeps us all alive, that subtle but relentless movement is what animates our body and mind, that tiny little place in the middle of the chest can hold such a big repertoire of emotions. It is a very profound experience to feel someone else's heart moving under my hand and that they are open enough for me to feel them in that intimate way. In that precious moment, there is no doubt that their heart is giving and I am receiving, even though it may seem like I am doing something for them. Their life prana is flowing into my hand and a motherly feeling arises in me, a quality of being nurturing and protective toward them. I like having that feeling, but I can't conjure it up; it's their opening that gives rise to my genuine response.

According to Jonathan Haidt, Ph.D. and recipient of the John Templeton Positive Psychology Prize (which encourages scientific study of qualities such as optimism, courage, compassion, and generosity), the warm feeling that naturally arises when we see another person doing a good deed, or learn of acts of kindness and courage, is called "elevation."

Haidt says not only does this arise in us when we recognize others' heartfelt actions and intentions, but that elevation is contagious. When we feel inspired by goodness, we begin to open up and feel more loving, appreciative, and compassionate. Haidt and his associates have been able to scientifically measure this feeling, experienced by some as tears, others as an expansion in the chest. They found that elevation acts on the vagus nerve, which regulates heart rate, and the warm-glow-in-the-chest feeling is actually the expression of a healthy change in heart rhythm. Opening to yourself and others might be scary, but it might also be good for you.

DISSOLVING BOUNDARIES

Tenzin Palmo, a Buddhist nun who grew up in Great Britain, lived in a cave in the Himalayan Mountains for twelve years. She was alone much of the time, and for the last three years, on a solitary retreat. In a dharma talk in New York City, she said, "Every person you meet is a chance to practice." After minimal human interaction for so many years, she ought to know! Every person is a chance to practice recognizing your tendency to respond through attraction or repulsion, to let go of that and to open to everyone you encounter, NO MATTER WHAT. To practice loving-kindness toward all beings. That takes a lot of commitment, but it is possible.

When I first met the Dalai Lama I was deeply inspired by his complete manifestation of kindness and humility. I recognized His Holiness as a bodhisattva and was moved to walk that same path. *Boddhi* means awake and *sattva* means being. Taking the bodhisattva vow is a way to pledge your life to working for the enlightenment of all beings. To put others first. The example of His Holiness was enough to change my life forever. As Dr. Haidt would say, I was elevated by the example of this beautiful monk.

Maitri, or loving-kindness meditation, is designed to help us remember that we are all connected, through our breath, our hearts, the pulsation of everything and everyone everywhere. Eido Roshi once said that he used to think he was being selfish by indulging in hours of zazen, meditating by himself for himself. But after thirty years of sitting, he realized that the transformative power of the practice radiated out from him, and others could feel that. Whatever you do affects everything else. Through our practice we all have the opportunity to help others, to elevate. On his deathbed, the Buddha said, "Make of yourself a light."

Is it possible that we can create world peace through yoga and meditation? I don't know, but, according to Chögyam Trungpa, "the way to rule the universe is to expose your heart." When the ebb and flow of our heart diminishes we feel separate from the vast world around us in which everything breathes, pulsates, expands, and contracts. Yoga, Buddhism, and all spiritual paths are a map showing the journey back to the heart of the universe, Big Mind, Great Spirit, the Source of all that is. And the heart of the universe is, of course, always within our own hearts, if only we can be brave enough to feel its movement.

Sometimes that bravery comes because we have no choice. My personal experience has been that when my heart is broken, just like my summer of tears, my boundaries start to soften and dissolve. When my father was told that he needed to have brain surgery, it was implied that he might not live long. Our small family, just my mom, dad, and me, was shaken and frightened. I have never before felt as alive as during the time of his surgery when we did not know what would happen. Everything was extremely intense and vivid. On the operating table, the doctors discovered that there was a serious brain infection but no tumor. Daddy would survive and be okay. During that period I practiced maitri/loving-kindness meditation for my father every day. When I first saw my dad's head with that big Frankenstein-like scar, my instinctive response was to touch my own head. I thought I was touching his head because in that moment,

I felt no separation between my body and his, between my head and his, between my heart and his.

MAITRI MEDITATION

Trungpa Rinpoche taught that one of the first elements of meditation posture was to take your seat with good "head and shoulders." If you are wakeful and present, you will naturally hold your head and shoulders in a dignified, uplifted way. If your head droops, it lowers your vision and creates a self-centered reality, because you can't see anything else. This leads to paranoia about what's happening all around you, which is like animals who move through the world looking at the ground, mainly concerned with finding food and protecting themselves from predators and other dangers of their world. When we lift our heads, we can see other people and it takes the attention off ourselves, which naturally creates an opening in our heart.

If you practice this visualization, it will begin to change your relationship to everything and relax your boundaries. It can be challenging, so remember to be kind to yourself. Let your heart open on its own schedule.

Close your eyes and visualize three figures in front of you. One is a person that you love, one you hate, and one who is neutral.

Begin by focusing on the person you love. Maybe it is your parent or your child, someone you can say that you love unconditionally. Now feel your body filled with a warm liquid, the milk of compassion. Let that warm white milk form a swirling ball in the middle of your chest. You can touch your chest, if you like. Open your heart and let the milk of compassion flow from your heart straight into the heart of this person that you care about so deeply. See their body filling up with warmth and light. Feel this connection.

Next, visualize a person that you do not like right now. It may be someone that is giving you difficulty or acting unkindly toward you. You may think of them as an enemy. Choose someone that is involved in your personal life rather than a historical or political figure that you have never met. If you find it impossible to do this exercise with your enemy, that's okay. Even just considering doing it is a start. Do not push yourself. If you can do it, then once again, imagine yourself full of warm, wonderful liquid as if your heart were circulating compassion through your veins. Let this milk come together in a soft ball in your heart, open the door of your heart, and pour this liquid into the heart of your difficult person. Know that they suffer, too, and give them the milk of compassion straight from you to them. See their whole body filling with it and imagine how they might feel better and benefit from that transformation.

Now think about a person in your life that is a stranger to you. Try to choose someone that you see on a regular basis but never really pay much attention to, perhaps the clerk at the cleaner's, the gas station attendant, or the street person who sleeps on the library steps. Visualize them as clearly as possible. Feel your body being filled with the milk of compassion and notice how it feels to be 100 percent compassionate. Let the feeling fill your heart so completely that you naturally open and let the milk of compassion flow straight into the heart of that stranger. See how your intention for loving-kindness can fill another person with loving-kindness as well. Notice what it is like to do this for a stranger, remembering that you are a stranger to almost everyone else in the world.

Yoga Body

HEART OPENING SEQUENCES

Try to do the following heart opening sequences slowly, with a panoramic sense of physical and mental awareness. As the toxic tension in your muscles is released, your breath will naturally deepen, which, in turn, calms your nervous system. This rebalancing helps us feel more confident, and able to open to our environment, whether it is a loud city, a peaceful beach, or our own tense body.

You may want to go faster, push and pull, or withdraw altogether from the position. Unless you feel it to be an injurious situation, remain in each pose for as long as I have recommended. Staying in the asanas for an extended period allows you to begin to notice the impermanence of each sensation.

Just as in life, you may recognize your own tendency to run away, whether by spacing out, making mental notes, shifting the position, or going to the refrigerator. Come back to your breath. Notice how your body can seem to have both places and spaces. Watch the movie of your mind. Don't worry.

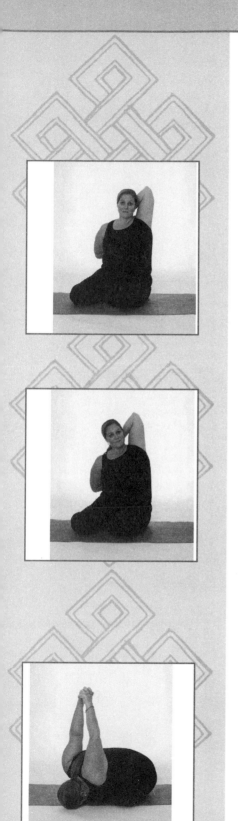

WARM-UP VINYASA FOR HEART OPENING

This is the same warm-up vinyasa as in the seated poses, only with arm variations that will open your chest and shoulders and upper back.

1. *Bharadvajrasana with Gomukhasana Arms* • Bharadvajra's Pose with Cowface Arms

Begin with both arms extended out to the sides from your shoulders. Externally rotate your left arm, lift it up, and bend it behind your head. Internally rotate your right arm, bend it, and reach your right fingers up to your left. If you cannot reach, use a belt. If you can reach, be aware of the quality of your touch—hold hands with yourself as you would like someone to hold hands with you.

2. *Bharadvajrasana with Side Bend Variation*

Exhale and bend to the right. Remember to keep your left hip connected to the ground. Sit on a cushion if it helps to balance your hips. After a breath or two, release your bottom arm to the floor. (Pictured on page 153.)

3. *Bharadvajrasana Twist*

Inhale back up to vertical, extending both arms up.

Exhale, twist to the left. (Pictured on page 153.)

4. Hip Opener/Forward Bend

Inhale back to center, and interlace your fingers behind your back.

Exhale, open one knee, and fold forward.

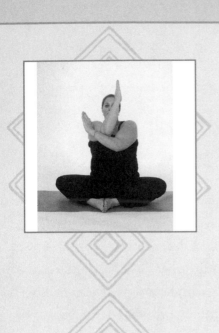

5. *Baddhakonasana* • Bound Angle or Cobbler's Pose with Garuda Arms

Inhale, sitting back up, and swing your arms around in front of you. At the same time that you bring the soles of your feet together, place your right elbow on top of your left and wrap your wrists. If your hands get contorted when you try to wrap your wrists, then place the backs of the hands against each other so you don't create more tension in your fingers and wrists.

Exhale here. Can you feel breath in between your shoulder blades? In backbending, even though we want to feel the strength of the shoulder blades firmly on our backs, we also want to allow the back muscles to broaden away from the spine.

Release your arms and shift your position to begin the second side.

Repeat side to side two to four times.

BEGINNER HEART OPENING SEQUENCE
Start with surya namaskar through the first downward-facing dog.

1. Psoas Opening Lunge

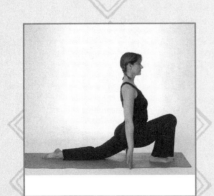

The psoas is a very long muscle that runs through the pelvis, connecting upper and lower and front and back bodies. If it is tight, it can create low back problems, restrict breathing, and make backbending very difficult. Step right leg forward to a lunge. Lower your back knee to the floor and let your sacrum melt forward. Let your right knee go as far forward as it can and still keep the right heel grounded. This will give you a good calf stretch.

In this position, move your thigh bones (femurs) to-

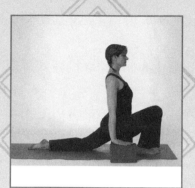

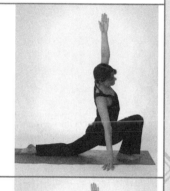

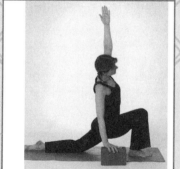

ward the muscles in the back of your thighs (the hamstrings). In other words, the front leg should be moving down toward the floor, but the back thigh should be energetically moving up and back, even though your knee is on the floor.

Lift your hip points and drop your tailbone, to minimize the sway of the lower back.

Lift your left arm up as you inhale. Exhale, and bend to the right. You can place your right hand on a block, or skim the floor with your fingertips. Inhale, back up.

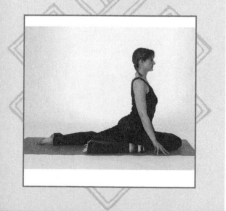

2. *Eka Pada Raja Kapotasana* • Pigeon

Place your palms on the floor and tuck your left toe under. Activate your back leg strongly enough that you can lift your hips up and shift your front leg into pigeon pose. Remember to use padding if one hip is off the floor.

Walk your hands forward and fold over your leg. Inhale, and curl your spine back up. Walk your hands back and come

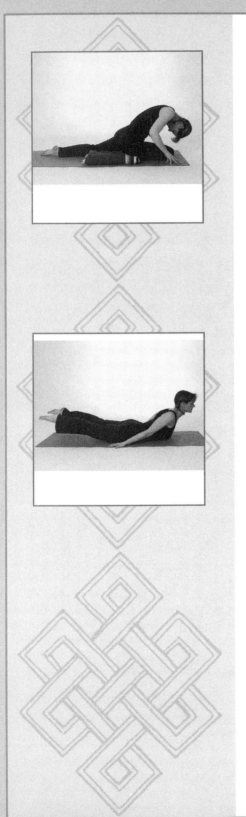

up onto your fingertips. This makes your arms longer so you can get more length in your torso.

Without using your hands, can you lift your back foot off the floor, even an inch?

Tuck your back toes under, straighten your back leg. Push your palms down and step back into downward-facing dog.

Repeat steps 1 and 2 to the other side before continuing on.

Inhale to plank and slowly lower yourself down onto your tummy.

3. *Salabasana* • Locust Mini Vinyasa

Place your forehead on the floor. Feet can be sitting bone distance apart.

Press your palms down and lift just your shoulders off the floor so your chest is open here. As if you were doing tadasana facing the floor.

Inhale, lift your chest, neck, and head. Keep some space open on the back of your neck.

Exhale, lift your legs up. Initiate this action from the top of your front thighs, just at your bikini line. Knees are straight, legs are strong, feet are pointed, but toes are soft.

Inhale, and lengthen out through your feet and the top of your head.

Exhale, lower everything back down to the floor.

Repeat this salabasana sequence two to four times.

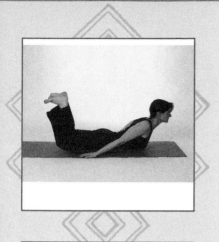

4. *Dhanurasana Preparation* • Bow Pose Prep with Bent Legs

Begin the same as with salabasana, except this time bend your legs. Flex your feet and try to maintain the position of ankles in line with knees in line with sitting bones.

Press your palms down and inhale, lifting your upper body and thighs up. Feel as if you could stand on the ceiling with your feet. Exhale, back down. Turn your head to the side to rest. Repeat two times.

5. *Ardha Dhanurasana* • Half Bow Pose

Lengthen your legs and place your forearms on the floor, elbows directly below shoulders. This is sphinx pose.

Bend your right leg and hold on to your ankle, not foot, with your right hand. If you can't reach it, use a belt.

Press your left hand down and straighten your left arm. If this is too much of a backbend, walk your left hand forward. Keep your left leg active, pressing it down and long.

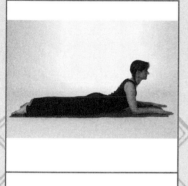

Exhale, and release back down. Try the other side.

6. *Ardha Urdhva Dhanurasana* • Half Wheel

Lying on your back, place your heels in line with your sitting bones. Press the soles of your feet and the palms of your hands down as you lift your torso up. Experiment with trying to lift up from the belly button, not from the tailbone, which will allow you to create a nice backbending curve in your spine.

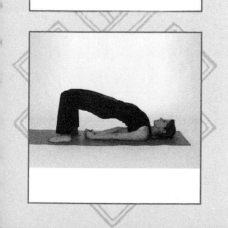

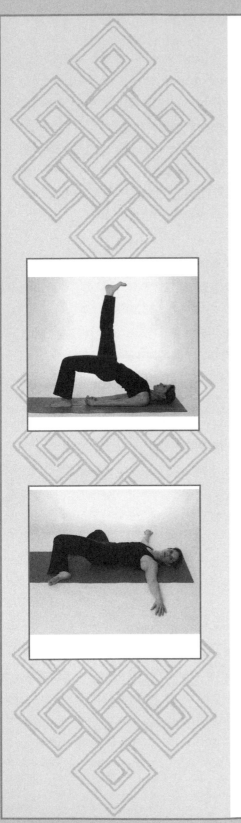

Once you are up, you can rock from side to side, rolling your shoulders under. Interlace your fingers behind your back. Can you feel how the shoulder blades underneath you help open the chest without it getting too hard? Relax your throat and jaw.

On an exhale, unclasp your hands and lower down, letting your sitting bones be the first thing that touches down. Repeat two times.

7. *Ardha Urdhva Dhanurasana Variation* • Half Wheel with One Leg Up

One more time, lift up into half wheel. This time, as you inhale, bring your right knee into your chest. Exhale, and extend your right foot straight up to the ceiling. Really push down with the left foot. Feel your arms grounding down, too. Replace your right foot to the floor. Do the other leg. Release your arms from underneath you and rest down.

8. Windshield Wipers

With bent knees, place your feet as wide apart as your mat. Let your knees fall to the right and left, slowly going back and forth like windshield wipers on the slowest setting. Your face can go in the opposite direction as your knees.

Can you feel the shape of your back, sacrum, skull, as you rock back and forth?

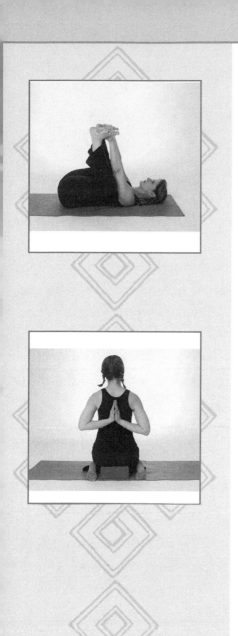

9. *Dead from Natural Causes Bug Asana a.k.a. Ananda Balasana*
  • Happy Baby Pose

Bring your knees toward your armpits and hold on wherever you can honestly reach and still keep length in your spine. If your bum is lifting up off the floor, hold on to your inner thighs, rather than your feet. Move your breath into the broadness of your back.

INTERMEDIATE HEART OPENING SEQUENCE

1. *Virasana with Reverse Anjali Mudra* • Hero's Pose with Reverse Prayer Hands

Come into this asana like this: Bring your knees together and your feet apart. Lean forward and place your head on the floor. Reach around behind you and pull the flesh and skin of your calves straight back toward your feet, away from the back of your knees. As you start to sit down, try to press your calf muscles flat, which sort of divides the calf muscles in two, creating a little ditch for your thigh to sit in.

This is a great opportunity to use props. Most all of us need to sit on something to be in balance here. If your sitting bones do touch the floor, you still may need to sit on something if your pelvis is tucking under.

This position will help to broaden the sacrum as well as deepen the groins.

Deepen your breath and feel the in-breath drop all the way to the groins.

Exhale the breath up and out your heart. Find lift and breath in the inside of the side ribs.

If you cannot do prayer hands, try doing it with the fingertips pointing down. Or you can hold on to your elbows or wrists.

You can stay for a while, even five minutes or more.

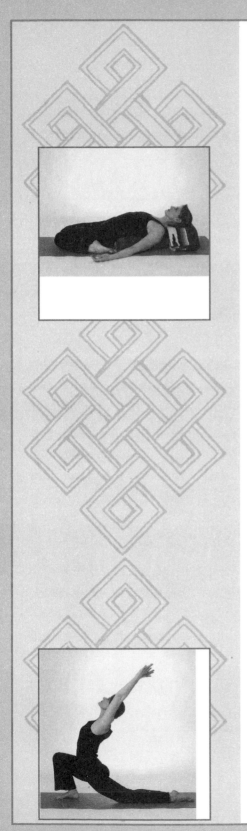

2. *Supta Virasana* • Reclining Hero's Pose

Both supta virasana and virasana are real opportunities to practice loving-kindness to yourself. This is a big psoas and quadriceps opener and you may feel a lot of sensation in those areas and in your knees and low back. Don't bully your way through these poses. Accessorize and cultivate patience, compassion, and curiosity. You will get the best results that way.

Your padding for supta virasana can be like a waterfall, so your forehead is higher than your chin is higher than your chest is higher than your knees.

Stay here for a while but not too long. You can decide.

Slowly sit up, by putting weight on your elbows, then shifting forward more and more. Take your time.

3. *Adho Mukha Svanasana* • Downward-Facing Dog

Shift your weight onto your hands and slowly lift your hips into downward-facing dog (page 104). Move symmetrically.

Stay here for about five breaths. You can also tread your feet in place as if you were riding a bike. Aren't these interesting sensations?

4. Psoas Opening Lunge with Chest Opener

Step your right leg forward into a low lunge. Hook your thumbs and inhale, to lift your arms up next to your ears. Keep your ears in line with your arms so your neck doesn't get squished. Take your time and several breaths to open the chest more and more. A very high lifted backbend action.

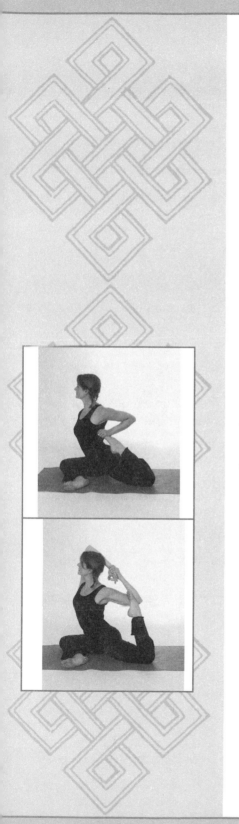

Let go of your thumbs and backstroke your arms. Place your palms on the floor on either side of your front foot. Tuck your back toes under, lengthen that leg, and lift your hips, shifting your right leg into pigeon pose.

5. *Eka Pada Raja Kapotasana* • Pigeon

First take a check of your alignment—back leg straight back, hips balanced (use a cushion if you need it), hips and nipples pointing straight ahead.

Then go ahead and walk your hands forward and fold over. (Pictured on page 158.)

Inhale and come on back up.

6. Full Pigeon Preparation

Bend your left leg behind you and hold on to it with your left hand. Gently draw your left foot toward your buttock for a quadricep stretch. If this is workable for you, then you can try to hook your left elbow around your ankle, coming into a variation of full pigeon.

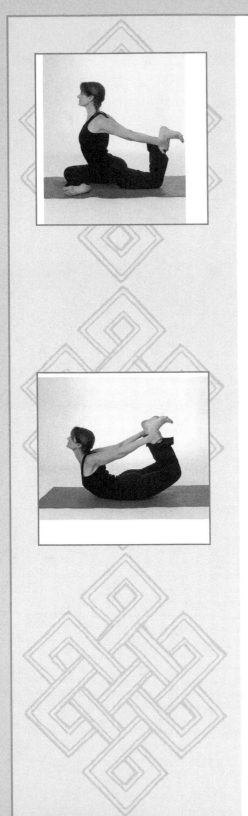

7. Pigeon with Half Bow

Hold on to the ankle of your bent back leg with both hands. Make an action with that back leg as if you were trying to straighten it. At the same time, soften the space behind your heart.

Release and step into downward-facing dog.

Repeat the psoas opening lunge, pigeon, and pigeon variations (4-7) to the other side before continuing on.

From your second downward-facing dog, inhale to plank pose and lower down through chaturanga, all the way to the floor.

8. *Dhanurasana* • Bow Pose

Bend both legs and hold on to your ankles. Check the alignment of ankles in line with knees in line with sitting bones. Reach your ankles back and let that action lift you up into bow pose.

It is important that you don't overwork the buttock muscles in backbending because it can jam up your lower back. Use your legs more than your bum.

Feel the inner thighs relating to each other. Imagine the outer thighs moving toward each other.

Release down. Turn your head to the side and rest. Repeat three times.

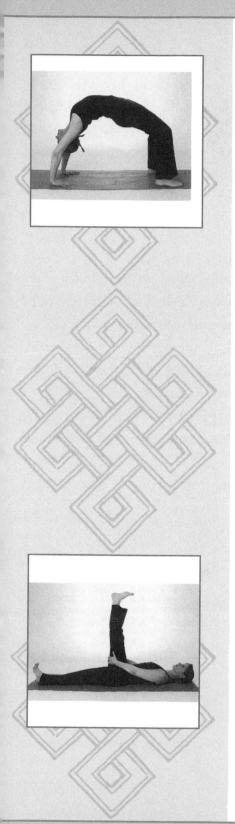

9. *Urdhva Dhanurasana* • Wheel Pose

In this pose, it is particularly important to recall the three parts of a pose: getting into it, being there, and coming out. Take care to align your wrists with your shoulders, elbows directly above, not rolling away from each other. If your elbows won't go straight up, turn your fingers out toward the sides of the mat, which will give you more external rotation in the arms and increased mobility in the shoulders. Don't lose this alignment on the way down.

Make sure the legs are aligned evenly—knees and toes pointing straight ahead—and maintain this on the way up and down.

Just as in half wheel, try to lift the navel up as you press your palms and feet down.

If you can't get up, try placing your hands on blocks. Do what you can and don't worry or get aggressive. This is just another thing to work on. You cannot open your heart by being pushy.

After three wheels, place your feet apart the width of your mat, turn your feet in pigeon-toed, and let your knees fall together. Arms open and rest. Breathe into your back.

10. *Supta Padangusthasana*

Instead of a hamstring stretch or forward bending action, we will do this pose in a way that neutralizes the spine after backbending.

Lift your right leg up and hold on to the back of your right thigh. Press your thigh into your hand, finding length in the torso. Reach the back of your left thigh down into the floor. Look for tadasana within this shape.

Change legs and do the other side.

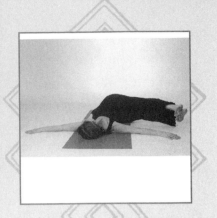

11. *Jathara Parivartanasana*

Lift both legs up on an exhale. Inhale, and then again on an exhale, lower them to the left, hovering about two inches from the floor. Slide your belly to the right. Press the back of your hands firmly down. Stay here for a couple of breaths, and then exhale the legs back up and go to the other side.

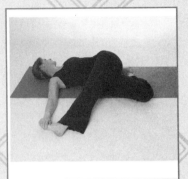

12. Busby Berkeley Variation

With the legs straight up again, lower just the right leg down to the floor. Hold on to your left ankle with your right hand or a belt. Exhale and lower your left leg across your body over to the left. Bend your right leg underneath you and take hold of that ankle with your left hand. Try to keep both shoulders flat on the floor.

After a few breaths, release the bottom leg, lift the left leg straight up. Bring the right leg up to meet it and then slowly lower the left leg down. Twist to the other side. After you finish that side, bring both legs up and slowly lower them straight down to the floor.

ADVANCED HEART OPENING SEQUENCE

As you move through these challenging poses and fancy variations, try to stay connected to your felt experience and less to getting anywhere. This is all about opening and it takes being strong to do that. Be curious and kind to yourself as a way to practice being that way to others. That is the most advanced variation of all.

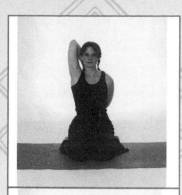

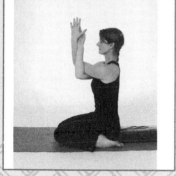

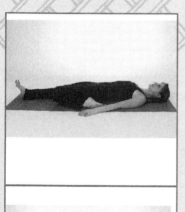

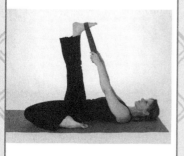

1. *Virasana with Gomukhasana and Garuda Arms* • Hero's Pose with Cowface and Eagle Arms

Sit in virasana for one to five minutes or more. In both of these arm variations, explore the breath through the chest, upper back, shoulders, neck. Drop your tongue to the bottom of your mouth and soften the space between your eyes. Watch your thoughts and emotions arise and pass while you stay steady in your seat.

Who is the hero of this pose? Possibly, it is you, in a similar way that we can be a warrior when we are brave, open-hearted and grounded enough to sit with whatever comes up for us in this pose right now.

Make sure to do arm positions to both sides.

2. *Supta Ardha Virasana* • Reclining Half Hero's Pose

Shift your weight to the left and, keeping your right heel close to your right buttock, bring the leg around and straighten it. Slowly lower down, first onto your elbows, then all the way onto your back. You can certainly use blankets under your back, as you did in supta virasana, to make this pose be habitable for you.

You can keep the right leg straight, or for some people it is more manageable at first to bend it and place the foot on the floor. You may find this whole sequence very intense. Take a long-term view and give yourself plenty of time with this asana—decades, even.

If you choose to extend your right leg up and then out to the side, you can use a belt around your foot. As you take the right leg out to the side, you can place a block under the thigh

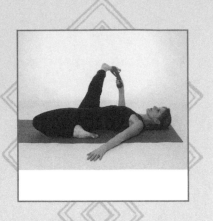

or calf so that you can stay there for a few breaths while keeping your pelvis balanced.

Inhale, and lift the leg back up. Bend the right knee and place the foot on the floor. Slowly sit up in half virasana.

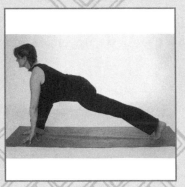

3. Lunge

Shift your weight forward onto your hands and step your left leg, the one that has been bent for so long, slowly straight back into a long lunge. Stay here for several breaths, letting the blood flow through your left leg freely.

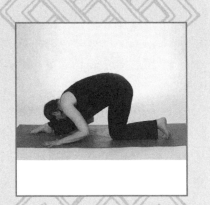

4. Forward Bend

Shift hips back and fold over front leg, as if you were in a one-legged pascimottanasana (Pictured on page 165.)

After several breaths here, inhale up.

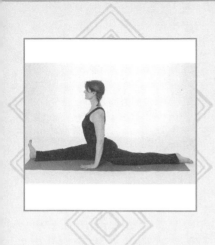

5. *Hanumanasana* • Splits

Keep the back toes tucked under at first, so you can really keep that leg straight, parallel, moving directly back, and actively extending through the four corners of the foot. Use blocks under each hand to help you maintain the reference point of tadasana even if your hips are above the floor.

This pose is named for a monkey god who was known for leaping and laughing.

Can you lift the corners of your mouth a little bit here? Don't work toooooo hard—remember, it's only yoga, after all.

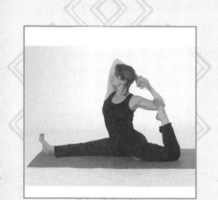

6. *Hanumanasana* • Splits with Leg Variations

If your hips are grounded on the earth and your spine is lifted, you can try to lift your back foot up and take hold of it like we did in the pigeon pose variations in the intermediate sequence. Holding it in the crook of your elbow or with both hands are options.

Release your leg and place your palms on either side of your front foot. Use your inhalation to help you lift your hips up so high that you can slide your front leg straight back into downward-facing dog.

Tread your feet in place as if riding a bike and then jump forward, landing lightly on your shins. Organize your legs into half virasana on the other side and repeat this sequence from there up to this point (2–6).

7. *Arm Preparations for Eka Pada Raja Kapotasana* • Full Pigeon

From downward-facing dog, bring your right knee into your chest, externally rotate your right thigh, and sit down in pigeon pose. Extend both arms up next to your ears and rotate

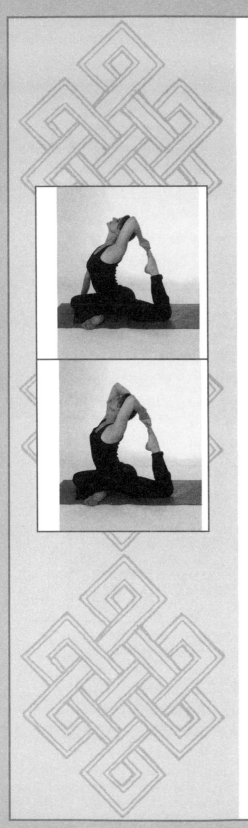

them out so that the palms face back. This is a good place to stay and work for a while. If you want to continue, bend your elbows and walk your fingertips down your shoulder blades, keeping a sense of lift in the back ribs and softness in the front ribs.

8. *Eka Pada Raja Kapotasana* • Full Pigeon
Place your palms down and bend your left leg. Hold on to it with your left hand. You can catch the outside of the foot with your very externally rotated left hand. Bring your hand and foot close to your shoulder, then dip your left elbow down, forward, and up. Now you are halfway into full pigeon.

Lift your right arm up next to your ear and reach back to find your left foot. You may find your left wrist and you can hold that and eventually walk your hand down to your foot. You can also practice this by looping a belt over your left foot and holding the belt with both hands overhead.

Think of your back being broad and moving the breath there. Feel the circle you are making with your body. Try to cultivate equal awareness and effort in all parts of your body.

Gently release out of this pose and step into downward-facing dog. Pedal your feet and then try the other side.

9. *Urdhva Dhanurasana* • Wheel Pose
From downward-facing dog lower onto your belly and roll over. Establish your alignment preparation for wheel. (Pictured on page 191.) On an inhale, press down into the earth to lift up. Can you let this be a sensuous opening, as if you were doing the first big stretch and yawn of the morning? Feel how the strength of your arms and legs allows your chest to be open. What does it feel like to be that vulnerable? Liberating, scary, a little of both?

Practice as many as ten wheels, being mindful that your elbows and knees point away from each other all the time. Let your head drop down as you lift up and keep length and softness in the next. You can do three wheels, with a rest in between each one. Then try doing the fourth, fifth, and sixth on one breath each, i.e., inhale up and exhale down, right away inhale up and exhale down and again right away inhale up and exhale down. This is almost like doing push-ups in wheel pose and will help you develop strength as well as spunk. Rest.

Here are some other fun wheel experiments: Try doing one of the wheels for a full minute without hardening or bulldozing through the experience. Try doing only one wheel for three minutes. Try to do one wheel in your mind, but really visualize it fully, with correct breathing and alignment. Then do it in your body and see if you learned anything from your psychic wheel.

10. *Eka Pada Udhva Dhanurasana* • One-Legged Wheel Pose
In wheel, lift one leg straight up to the ceiling. Other side.
Come down and rest.

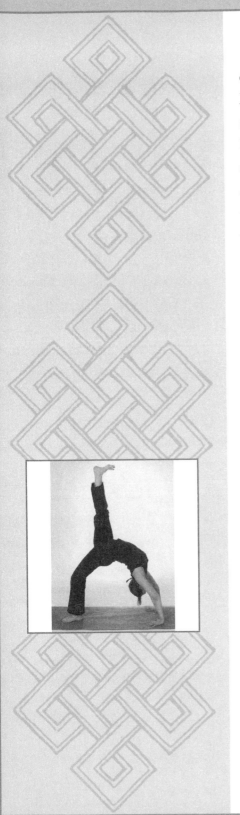

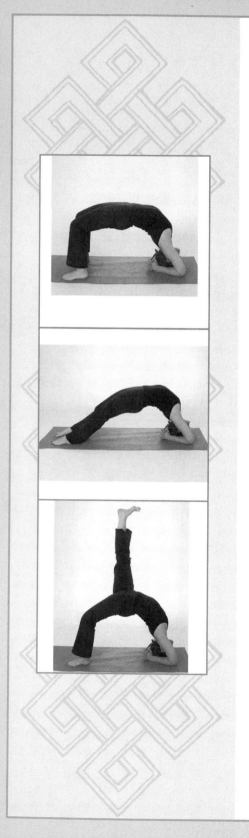

11. *Dwi Pada Viparita Dandasana* • Two Feet Inverted Stick Pose

From wheel pose preparation, inhale and lift up just to the top of your head. Interlace your fingers around your head, like a headstand. Begin to walk your feet out. Reach into the floor with the four corners of the feet to help open the chest and prevent the legs from rolling out. Press down with your forearms. You can practice doing this without straightening your legs, too. You can also try a one-leg-up variation.

Release by walking your feet back in, placing your hands next to your shoulders, lifting up to the crown of your head. Then tuck your chin into your chest and come down on your shoulders.

Finish with the same counterposes as in the intermediate sequence:

12. *Supta Padangusthasana*
(Pictured on page 191.)

13. *Jathara Parivartanasana with Bent Knees*

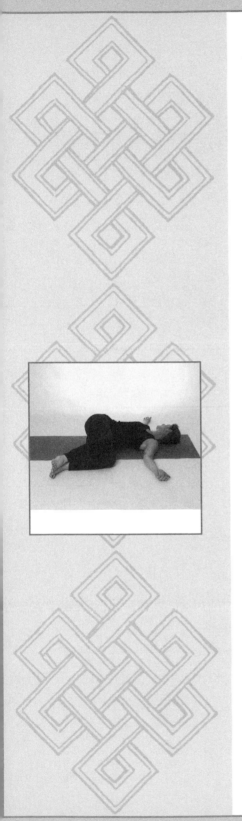

TEN

TOPSY-TURVY WORLD

Inversions

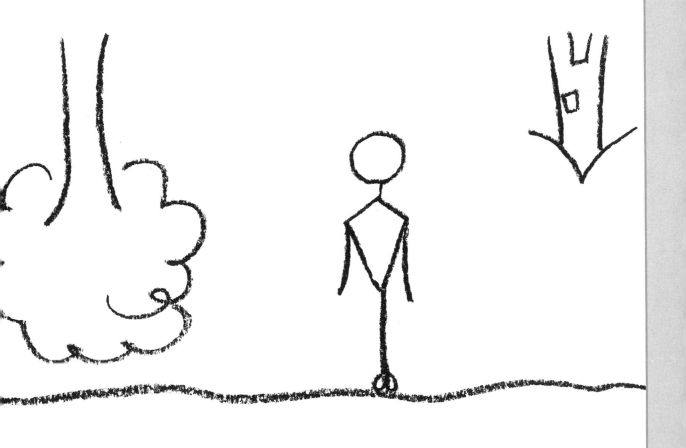

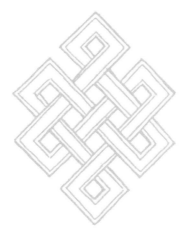

Buddha Mind

FREE FROM FIXED MIND

Inversions are the secret weapon of yoga. Other than gymnasts, how many people do you know who turn upside down on a regular basis? Even gymnasts who walk and stand on their hands usually flip onto their feet after a few moments and continue with their routine. Not yogis. We go up and stay up. An advanced yogi might even practice a headstand or shoulder stand for over thirty minutes and find the experience to be one of well-being, equanimity, and repose.

Part of the potency of inversions stems from the rebalancing that occurs between the lower and upper parts of our energy body. In yoga anatomy, the downstairs part of our body contains the apana vayu, and upper part contains the prana vayu. The apana vayu, or downward-moving wind, relates to the feminine aspect of our energetic being associated with earth and nature. It is located below the diaphragm, travels in an earthward direction, and affects abdominal organ functions such as digestive and reproductive issues. This is the opposite of the prana vayu, the upward-moving wind energy that affects respiration and heart rate and is associated with the masculine aspect of conceptual mind and sky.

Because we are usually standing or sitting, our apana vayu circulation slows down or gets stuck in our lower regions, where it becomes dull. And because we exercise too little, but talk and think too much, our prana vayu gets overstimulated and overused. We depend on our mental abilities to understand our world and less on our sensations and intuition. Inversions allow us to reverse the dominance of our conceptual mind over our intuitive mind, and our fixed notions over our direct experience.

Yoga asana practice offers us many opportunities to establish balance in our physical situation—right and left, front and back. But the deeper effect of letting go of fixed mind, of seeing the world from a different perspective, of calmly abiding in a topsy-turvy upside-down world—that may be the most profound benefit of yoga.

Trungpa Rinpoche called this "suddenly free from fixed mind." Our ideas and opinions, whether they are regarding beauty, politics, or health, are not solid. Our perspective, as if looking out from the center of a circle, is not solid. It is just one point of view. Up is not always up. Down is not always down. When we reverse our visual field, our base of physical support—not to mention our idea of what is sane, healthy, or fun—we are taking a courageous step toward the willingness to simply dance with energy without attaching to labels or preconceived notions.

Buddhism expresses this idea in a teaching called the Heart Sutra, which begins with the phrase, "Form is emptiness; emptiness also is form." In *An Introduction to the Buddha and His Teachings,* the Nalanda Translation Committee comments, "Form is emptiness means that all phenomenal forms—trees, pencils, shouts, moods, etc.—as they really are, are empty of all the concepts by which we grasp them and fit them into our world, empty of all we project upon them."

This means that we can learn to relate to things as they are, not as we wish they were, or as they used to be, but how they are right now . . . and now . . . and now as they keep changing. When we are stuck on only one way for things to be, then we are truly stuck. Then when our world shifts dramatically—which it will, through the death of a loved one, a change of employment, even falling in love—we will find that we are thrown for a loop because we have committed to our world being only one way and that way will have vanished. Turning upside down is practice for this. It offers us a fresh perspective. When one can remain in this environment with calm abiding, it is the beginning of the ability to stay centered when your world turns upside down.

OVERCOMING FEAR

One of the most common mental obstacles to doing inversions is fear. Some people are afraid that their arms cannot hold them up. Some are afraid of new sensations such as lifting their feet off the ground. Some are simply afraid of failing. It is worth taking the time to look at your fear and determine how much of it is habitual.

A few years ago some of my yoga students invited me to go scuba diving. They were so insistent on showing me the beautiful undersea world that I finally had to admit to them that I was afraid to swim in the ocean. Luckily, one of the women in the group was a psychotherapist experienced in helping people overcome fears, and she offered to meet with me the next afternoon.

I was both skeptical and hopeful. Many people have tried to teach me to swim in waves, to coax me out into the ocean, to talk me out of the fear that grabs me the minute I see a wave coming toward me. Sometimes I can get past the fear a little bit, but it usually takes a whole summer, and then by the next summer I am completely paralyzed again.

My husband's diagnosis was that something had traumatized me when I was young, but I said, "No, I have just always been like this." When he met my mother he asked her about it and she said right away, "Oh, yes, Cyndi almost drowned when she was twelve. She got battered about by big waves, thrown against some rocks, and was quite frightened. After that, she would only swim in the pool." When my mom told us that, I remembered the incident clearly, but until then it was evidently only an unconscious, cellular—but powerful—memory.

The therapist asked me to recall that day, and then asked if there were any other water issues in my memory. To my surprise, several water traumas surfaced, mostly incidents that had occurred when I was young. Until that moment all of these memories existed as a solid wall of fear that did not allow me to swim in the ocean, or even a flowing river, without my knowing why.

As I continued to recall these experiences out loud, I realized that the fear responses I'd had back then might have been natural for a young and extra-small girl. But I'm grown up now and no longer a fearful person. I have confidence in my physical strength, my innate intelligence, and my ability to make safe choices. It was suddenly obvious to me that I don't have to respond to water the way I did when I was twelve years old, any more than I would make timid choices about anything else based on my twelve-year-old mind.

How liberating! And it worked. The next day I went on a sailboat ride, with a life jacket on, of course, and I jumped into the middle of the deep blue sea and swam around with my friends. It was fun and only a little bit scary. This experience was profound for me and I carried away two things that have been helpful in every way: 1) the mind is a powerful obstacle; 2) I don't need to be afraid of fear.

When one of my good friends first started studying yoga with me she told me she could only watch in amazement as, in her words, "I floated like a butterfly up into a headstand." She said, "I can't imagine ever standing on my head!" Since she was strong, coordinated, and had good alignment, I realized that lack of imagination was her biggest stumbling block. Totally reversing your body in space is far beyond the wildest dreams of many of us. It is out of the question for most people who do not think that reversing their gravitational relationship to the earth is a good thing anyway, and certainly not their idea of fun, or anything other than nuts!

Why is it only good to stand on your feet? Why can't we stand on our hands and use our arms like legs? Why do we always stand on the floor? When we completely reverse our body and our relationship to gravity, we threaten the ground of these ideas. When we are able to remain inverted with calmness and curiosity we begin to expand the notion of what is real, fixed, and solid.

One student did a headstand for the first time and thought it was fun. He told me, "Wow, it looks like everyone is stuck to the ceiling!" A yogi is continually expanding their definition of what fun is, too!

Many people do not think of themselves as imaginative, but we are all braver and more creative than we think. How many things can you do now that you never thought you could or would even want to do? Get married, own a business, have children, run a marathon, care for a dying relative, bake a perfect soufflé, practice yoga. When you were twelve months old you couldn't walk, but you didn't stop trying. You saw other people doing it and you gave it a try. Even though you fell down a lot, you kept going and now you do it without a second thought.

One of the first baby steps to doing inversions is imagining that you can. You can actually practice asanas—or anything physical—this way. When I was a professional dancer we rehearsed for hours and it was quite tiring. Eventually we discovered that we could rehearse in our heads at night and actually improve our performance without becoming exhausted. We actually made mistakes at the same point in our head-dance that we were making over and over in rehearsal. We could mentally review the mistake, correct it, and by going over it several times clearly in our minds, we found that when we got back to rehearsal we had repatterned ourselves and did not make that mistake anymore.

I have heard that Phil Jackson, former coach of the Chicago Bulls and now coach of the L.A. Lakers, as well as a Zen Buddhist, uses similar visualization techniques to train his winning basketball players, like Michael Jordan. This can be applied to anything, as John Lennon suggested: "Imagine all the people living life in peace. . . ." If everyone imagined that, what might happen?

The second thing I learned from my water breakthrough was that a healthy dose of fear can be just that—healthy. The therapist asked me what my ideal ocean experience would be and I said that I wished I could be like my friends who run, madcap and joyous, into the ocean. When they hit the water it tumbles them around like a washing machine and they bounce up laughing! She told me that even those people who are having a blast in the waves have a tiny bit of fear—not habitual fear that paralyzes, but just genuinely sharp enough to keep them paying attention. Nobody with any intelligence at all would go swimming in the ocean without an edge tuned in to the constant changes in their environment. In fact, that is part of the exhilaration and satisfaction. The vibrancy of being completely alive, not knowing what is coming and responding fresh to every single moment. Can you be brave enough to let your body and intuition guide your choices as much as your well-informed brain does?

YOGA BODY

KING AND QUEEN ASANA

The physical benefits of inversions are so many and so powerful that headstand and shoulder stand are considered the king and queen, or father and mother, of all yoga asanas. All asanas tone and build muscle strength but only weight-bearing poses, such as standing poses, develop bone mass. Inversions, and asanas that prepare for inversions, are considered to be standing poses—you just happen to be standing on something besides your feet. These weight-bearing asanas will develop muscle and bone density in the wrists, arms, chest, upper back, and shoulders, which is where most fractures occur due to osteoporosis.

In addition to the effects on the outer form, there are vital health benefits happening internally, as well. Sirsasana—headstand—stimulates the pineal and pituitary glands in the brain, the master glands of the endocrine system which control chemical balance throughout the entire body. Salamba sarvangasana—shoulder stand—stimulates the thyroid and parathyroid glands, which regulate metabolism.

Inversions improve circulation in the lower body, relieving strain and fatigue in the legs and feet, draining fluids, and massaging inner organs aiding in digestion and elimination. They act as a natural face-lift by improving blood circulation to the muscle and skin cells of the face. Both melatonin and seratonin are stimulated, which aids in sleep and relaxation. Mental clarity and concentration is honed through the challenge of inverting your physical position.

All these benefits make it worth the time it takes to learn inversions. You may still feel like this part of the practice is not for you, but remember, everything changes all the time. Did you ever know someone from a distance—maybe a coworker or somebody you went to school with—whom you could just tell from what you observed that you didn't like at all. Then, through circumstance, you ended up getting to know them and now they are one of your dearest friends. This could happen with inversions. When you have been able to look your fear in the face, use your imagination, and develop strength in your arms, legs, and abdomen, you will be able to use your inversions as a way to relax your point of view whenever you need to clear your mind.

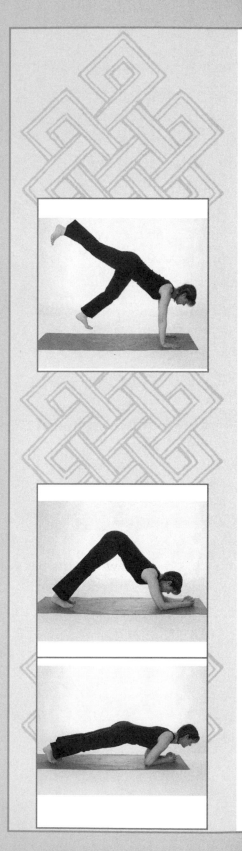

INVERSION SEQUENCES

BEGINNER INVERSION SEQUENCE

Begin with surya namaskar through to the first downward-facing dog.

1. *Adho Mukha Vrksasana Prep* • Handstand Preparation

Lift one leg up behind you, maintaining tadasana alignment in both legs. In other words, try not to roll open the top leg. Bend the bottom leg and jump up and down on it five times. Remember to always bend your supporting leg's knee at the beginning and ending of a jump. Change legs and jump up and down on that leg five times.

2. *Balasana* • Child's Pose Variation

Lower your knees to the floor. Keep the feet together but separate your knees wide apart. Walk your hands forward and lie down with either your forehead or your chin on the floor. After five breaths here, externally rotate your arms, rolling your thumbs up and then away from each other. Just see what's available to you. After a few more breaths, bend your elbows and place your palms on your shoulder blades. This external rotation and bending action is a big shoulder and triceps opener, which is helpful for both backbends and inversions.

Turn your palms down, tuck your toes under, and make your way back to downward-facing dog.

3. Dolphin

Keeping your legs active and sitting bones lifted, lower one forearm to the floor. Press that palm down to straighten the arm again. Other arm. Now try lowering both at the same time. Keep working on it and don't forget about how using your legs will help.

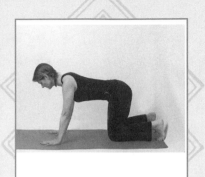

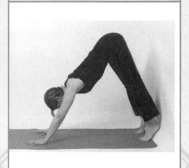

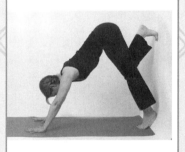

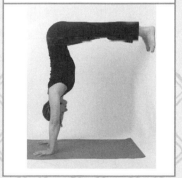

With both forearms down, organize your elbows directly below your shoulders, and interlace your fingers into a two-handed fist. Legs and body are as if in downward-facing dog.

Inhale, and as you exhale, lower your chin in front of your fist, inhale back up. This is called dolphin. Repeat this as many as ten times or as few as two. Rest and do more, eventually working up to fifteen dolphins.

Rest in child's pose.

4. *Adho Mukha Vrksasana Prep* • L-Shaped Handstand

Begin on your hands and knees with the soles of your feet facing right at the wall. Align your wrists directly below your shoulders and your knees below your hips. Without moving your hands or feet, lift your hips into downward-facing dog here. The first step then is to step onto the molding of the wall, if you have that. Next step is to place the right foot on the wall right behind your right hip. Press that foot into the wall as you push your hands down into the floor; this combo action will lift your hips.

All limbs must be very active here. Feet push into the wall, hands push into the floor, sitting bones reach up, up, up. After a breath or two, hop down and rest in child's pose. Work up to ten breaths. This could take a few months but isn't it amazing that you would even try to do this?

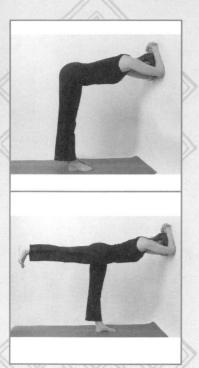

5. *Sirsasana Preparation* • Headstand Preparation

Touch your ears with your thumbs and then join your index fingers on the top of your head so it feels like you are wearing a Walkman. Where your fingers meet on the crown of your head is approximately where you will stand. Then interlace your fingers, align your elbows as wide as your shoulders, and place your forearms on the wall. Touch the headstand place you located on the crown of your head on the wall just behind your wrists and walk your feet out so you are in a 90-degree angle.

Inhale and lift your right leg straight back, as in warrior 3. Keep reaching the left sitting bone back as well and the forearms into the wall. Change legs. You can repeat each side a few times.

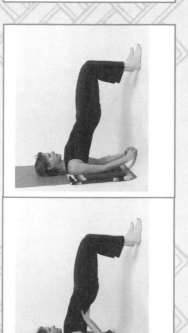

6. *Salamba Sarvangasana Prep* • Shoulder Stand Prep at Wall

Place a blanket near the wall and lie down on it so that your shoulders are at the edge of the blanket, your head and neck are off the blanket, and your sitting bones are at the wall. Bend your knees slightly, just enough to get your feet flat on the wall. Bend your arms and press your elbows down as you press your feet into the wall. Miraculously, your hips will lift right up! Roll your shoulders underneath you and interlace your fingers to open the chest. Then place your palms on your back and walk your feet, one at a time, up the wall. Activate your legs and reach through the four corners of your feet. This is similar to inclined plane pose. Relax your jaw.

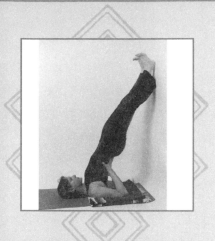

After about one minute, you can walk your feet down so your knees are bent; soften your hips and lower all the way back down.

INTERMEDIATE INVERSION SEQUENCE
Do intermediate surya namaskar to downward-facing dog.

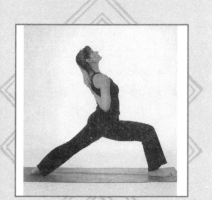

1. *Virabhadrasana 1 with Gomukhasana Arms* • Warrior 1 with Cowface Arms
Turn left heel down and step right foot forward, lifting up into warrior 1. Change arms to gomukhasana arm position.

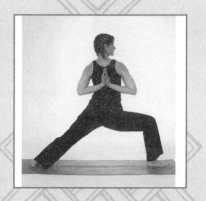

2. *Virabhadrasana 2 with Anjali Mudra* • Warrior 2 with Prayer Hands
When you exhale and open into warrior 2, keep the bottom arm where it was. Circle the top arm out of cowface and right around back to meet the right in reverse prayer hands, a nice chest opener.

Continue with surya namaskar: chaturanga, upward-facing dog, downward-facing-dog. Repeat 1 and 2 on the other side.

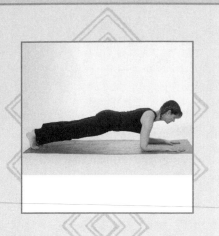

3. Forearm Plank

Inhale to plank and lower onto forearms. You will probably have to walk your feet back a bit so your shoulders are over your elbows. Activate your abs without gripping them. Shine energy out your feet and gaze slightly forward so your head doesn't hang in despair.

Lift one leg for three breaths. Then the other leg.

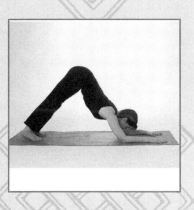

4. Downward-facing Puppy

Then lift hips into forearm downward-facing dog—called downward-facing puppy. From here lift one leg up as in downward-facing dog split, only on the forearms. Then the other leg up.

Rest in the wide-legged child's pose variation (described on page 210) with the arms extended forward and externally rotated. Move back into downward-facing dog and repeat 1–4 on the other side.

You can stop here or you can continue at the wall:

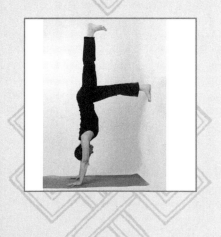

5. *Adho Mukha Vrksasana* • L-Shaped Handstand Variation

Lift up into L-shaped handstand. Slowly lift your right leg straight up toward the ceiling. Flex your foot strongly and tuck your head slightly so you can see your foot. If you cannot see your foot it means you are arching your back like a banana and your foot is too far toward the center of the room. If you are doing this correctly, you should be making the same shape as in warrior 3, only upside down. What does the world look like from this perspective? Count to three and change legs. Count to three. Replace the second leg on the

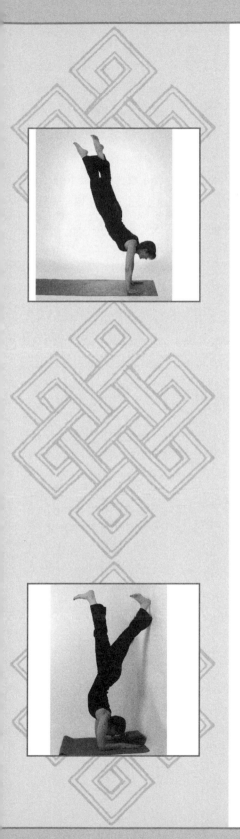

wall and then hop down and rest in child's pose. Build up to eight counts on each leg.

6. *Adho Mukha Vrksasana Prep* • Starting to Jump Up

Place your fingers about five inches from the wall in downward-facing dog. Walk your feet in, about four to five inches closer than usual, and shift your shoulders forward so they are over your wrists. Inhale and lift one leg, exhale and lower it halfway, inhale and kick it up at the same time that you jump up with the other leg. Practice this several times on each leg. Eventually you will go up.

It might be scary for you and that is not unusual. You can put a belt around your arms just above your elbows; this will give you some support. Take small jumps so you begin to get used to holding weight in your arms like that. Then a little bit bigger jump, also growing accustomed to the coordination that is involved. Over time you may find that you get more comfortable and confident, which will overtake your habit of fear and you'll fly up.

But in the meantime, take it slow and easy. There is no rush here. You will go up when you go up and not before that. Enjoy the ride.

7. *Pinca Mayurasana* • Forearm Stand with Props

It is helpful to use props this way: Hold your block between your hands and tie a belt around your arms just above your elbows. If your triceps, shoulder, upper back are tight, then roll up a blanket and place your elbows on it, with your palms off the blanket. This will help to open the angle of the upper arms and enable you to do this pose without creating a bananalike curve in your back as a compensation for tight upper body. It will also help you feel open in the chest.

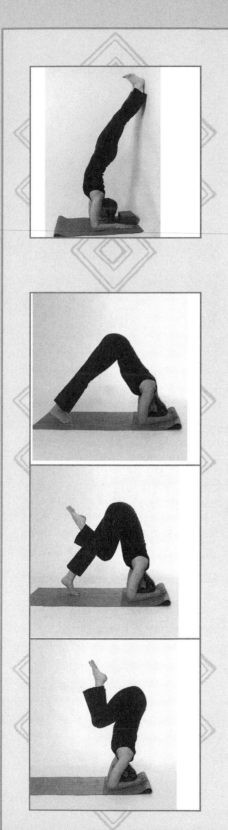

From this starting point, kick up the same way as in handstand. It is not as far so you will find that you might not need as much oomph to get there. Listen to the sound that your feet make when they contact the wall and you will know if you are working too hard.

Think of taking your feet up to the ceiling rather than the wall, so that your legs are long and active. This is how you begin to experience a sense of lightness and lift, and less panic. Rest in child's pose.

8. *Sirsasana* • Headstand

I recommend folding your mat in thirds. This is just the right amount of padding under your head and still quite firm. A blanket will generally be too soft and not supportive enough for your neck.

Place your two-handed fist on the floor and put the top of your head right in front of your wrists. Lift your hips as if in downward-facing dog. Check in with your shoulders and make sure your shoulder blades are firm on your back, not popping out. Make sure you strongly lift your biceps and triceps up your arm bones so your neck doesn't get smushed.

Walk your feet in a few inches. Keep reaching your sitting bones up.

At first: Stay for five breaths, then rest in child's pose.

Next: Bring one knee into your chest and count to five. Other knee for five counts and rest.

Finally: Bring one knee into your chest.

Hold it there tightly and lift the other knee into your chest. Find the wall with your feet and take your legs up. Keep your bum off the wall and the legs strong as if in tadasana. Steady your gaze and breath.

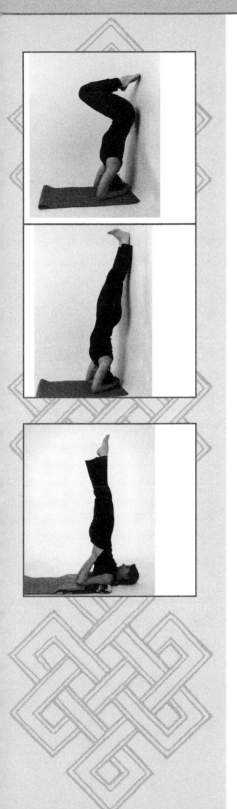

The first time you do this you should only stay up for about five breaths. When this feels comfortable, after several months, you can begin to increase it by fifteen seconds per week.

Rest in child's pose for five breaths and then in downward-facing dog for five breaths.

9. *Salamba Sarvangasana* • Shoulder Stand

Begin at the wall as in the salamba sarvangasana prep in the beginner sequence. Walk your legs up the wall and then, once at a time, take them off the wall. You can take just one leg off for a few breaths, replace it, and do the other leg. (See page 212).

With both legs off the wall, feel the spine moving into the chest to let it open without hardening. Soften the throat, jaw, eyes, breath. Say your name out loud and if you sound like a munchkin, try to broaden your collarbones, and let your chin and forehead fall back from your chest slightly. Try it again.

Stay here for five to ten breaths. Over time you can stay here for several minutes.

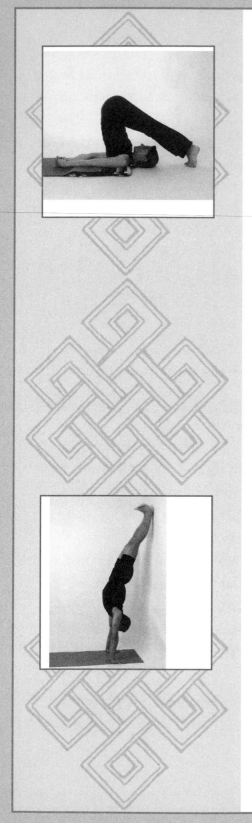

10. *Halasana* • Plough Pose

Keeping the sitting bones lifted, slowly lower your legs over your head. If your feet don't touch the floor, you can rest them on a chair or stack of books. If your feet do touch the floor you can take your hands off your back and rock side to side to reorganize your shoulders under you. Make sure, when you do that, that you are tucking the shoulders under and toward each other. You don't want to pull the shoulders down away from the ears here because it can over-stretch the skin and muscles of the neck. Stay here for five breaths.

Put your hands on your back and lift your legs back up to the wall. Roll down and rest.

ADVANCED INVERSION SEQUENCE
Place your mat far enough away from the wall so that if you stand in the top third of the mat, you can bend forward and your head will easily clear the wall.

1. *Adho Mukha Vrksasana Vinyasa* • Handstand Vinyasa

Stand at the two-thirds point of your mat and begin surya namaskar. When you get to downward-facing dog, kick up into handstand.

The wall is still right there so you don't have to worry about falling over backwards. Right before you lift up, visualize the air space just above your shoulders. Remember, at this point your shoulders should be stacked over wrists, so now your job is simply to stack your hips above that and your feet will follow if you keep your legs engaged. See that spot in your mind's eye and just place your pelvis there. You probably need less momentum than you think. Try finding out how

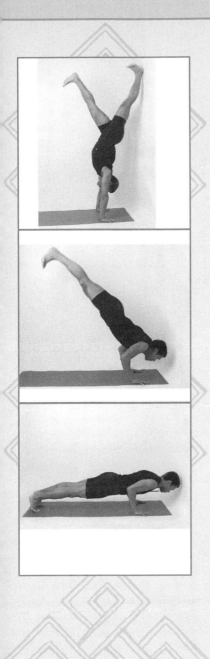

much effort is too little and that will help you find out how much is just exactly the precise amount required to get there.

You can also practice coming out of handstand into chaturanga by keeping one leg on the wall as long as possible. Slowly drag it down as you begin to bend your arms and eventually float down into chaturanga. It might not be as hard as you think.

Try this several times and change the kicking-up leg each time.

2. *Pinca Mayurasana Vinyasa* • Forearm Balance Vinyasa
You can also do the same sequence, lowering forearms down in downward-facing dog and lifting up into a forearm balance in the middle of the surya namaskar sequence. (See page 63).

Eventually you may be able to try these sequences without the wall! Start by creating that visualization.

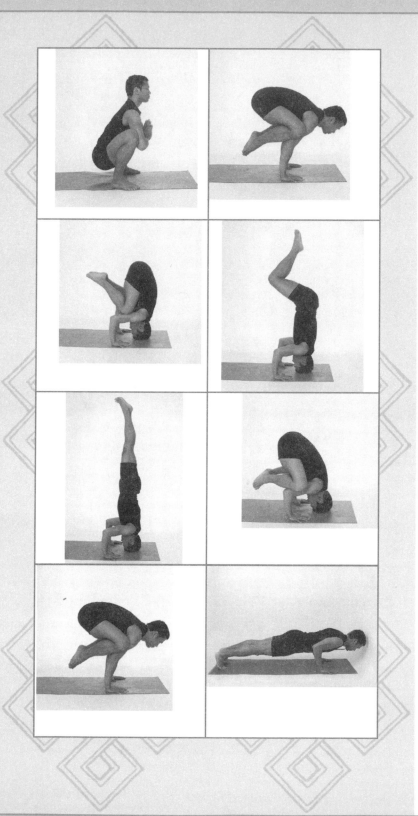

3. *Sirsasana Vinyasa* •

Headstand Vinyasa

Begin with surya namaskar to downward-facing dog, then jump feet to outside of hands in malasana preparation.

Come into crow pose. From crow pose, slowly bend your arms and keep your tummy lifted to lightly touch the crown of the head to the floor. Inhale your legs up into tripod headstand. Make sure your elbows are pointing straight back, as if they were in chaturanga. To come back down, keep the sitting bones lifted as you bend your knees and place them on the outsides of your upper arms. Think of lengthening the tailbone away from the top of the head rather than just trying to lift your head, which will probably make your hips drop and you fall out of crow. You might fall out anyway. Keep trying.

From crow pose, reach your shoulders and chest for-

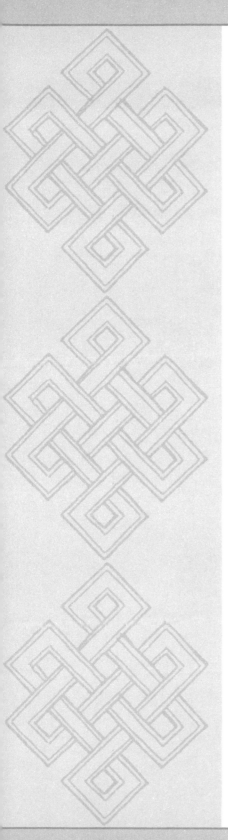

ward as you shoot your legs back, coming right into chatu-ranga, and continue to the end of surya namaskar.

4. *Salamba Sarvangasana Vinyasa* • Shoulder Stand Vinyasa

Inhale and rock up into shoulder stand.

Exhale, plough pose.

Inhale, roll down and right up into boat pose.

Exhale, cobbler's pose.

Inhale, tabletop.

Exhale, seated forward bend.

Inhale, sit up and bend your knees.

Exhale, twist right.

Inhale, center.

Exhale, twist left.

Repeat as many times as you like. Let the movement match the tempo of your own personal breathing pattern today.

You can try these variations if you want to stay in shoulder stand a little longer:

Bend your legs into baddhakonasana (cobbler's pose) or padmasana (full lotus). Place your hands on your knees with your arms straight.

Or, place your palms on your thighs with your legs wide apart in urdhva mukha upavista konasana (upward-facing open angle pose) and then if you feel steady, begin to bring the legs together, ending up in candle pose.

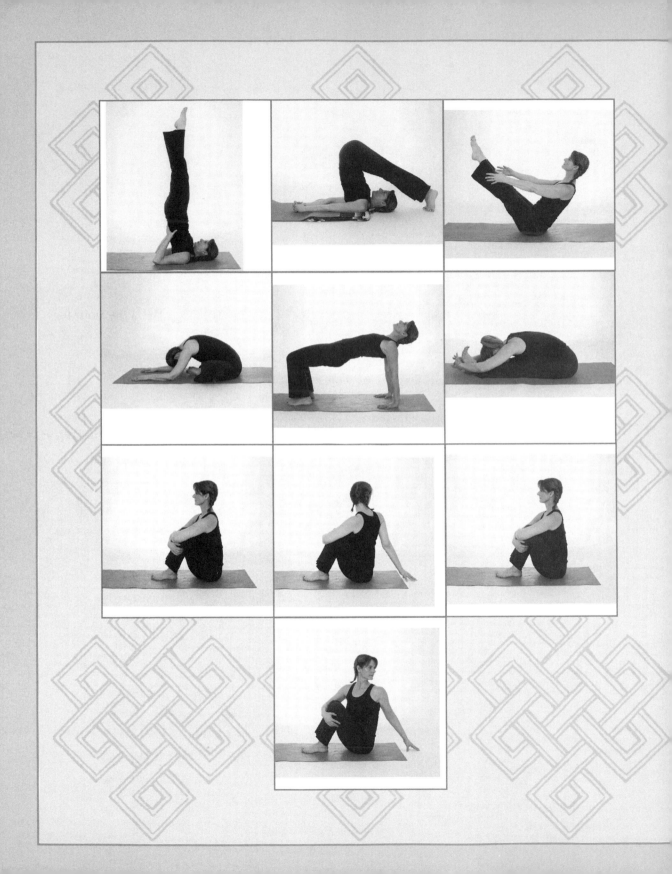

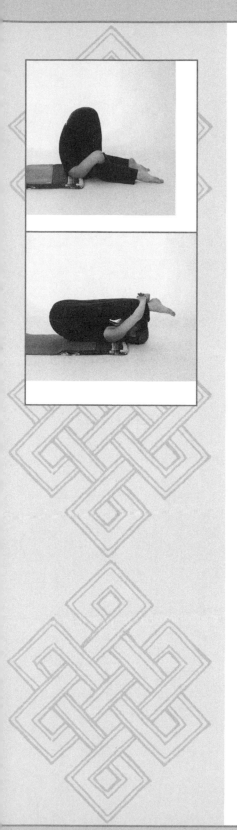

5. *Halasana and Karnepidasana* • Plough Pose and Crab Pose
Lower your legs into plough pose. Separate your legs and
bend your knees around your ears. You can wrap your arms
around the back of your knees, and place your palms over
your ears. A very internal pose. This is a very big stretch of
the entire back body so go slowly and gently. Give it time.

Place your hands on your back and use them as brakes to
control your roll down. If you are very loose in your hamstrings, you can wrap your arms around the back of your
thighs and slowly roll down through urdhva mukha pascimottanasana (upward-facing forward bend). Lower your legs
to the floor.

ELEVEN

HOW TO RELAX

Restorative Yoga

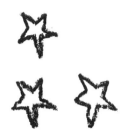

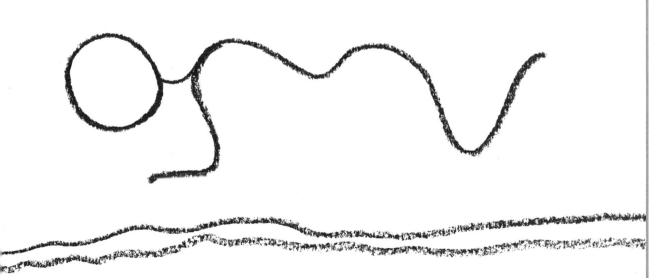

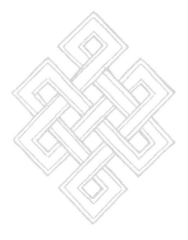

Buddha Mind

Only three weeks after I started high school, a very popular senior boy asked me out on my first date! I enjoyed the status promotion within my crowd of girl-friends, but secretly I was not looking forward to it. In fact, I was petrified. I had absolutely no experience with boys—no brothers, not even a next-door neighbor boy playmate. I simply didn't know anything about boys at all except that I was hoping a nice one would like me.

Although nobody who knows me now would ever believe it, I was so shy that during the entire evening I sat stock-still with my head tucked into my chest—unable to speak or even look at my date. I was utterly intimidated by his big-man-on-campusness. The worst moment of all was when, to my complete embarrassment, he touched my hand (!) and said "Relax." I had hoped he might think my quiet attitude was an expression of cool hipness, but obviously he could see that I was uncool and uptight. Each time he suggested I relax, I cringed more, until my whole being stayed tied up in an energetic contraction.

As suave as he was, neither my poor date nor I knew how to create a situa-tion that would allow me to let go and open up. Just as we can't find happiness by desperately wanting to be happy, or become enlightened by craving freedom from attachment, we can't force ourselves to be relaxed by saying, "Relax!"

For one thing, the very idea of not-doing as a way to make something happen is almost inconceivable to most of us. Society tells us to thrust forward with everything we've got in order to get anywhere in this world. Consequently, we become good at being active, but less good at being sensitive. When someone points and says, "Look!" we often find ourselves employing rapid eye-and-head movement to locate something that is right in front of us. It's the same for most of our other senses—we tighten our jaws and stick out our chin to hear a pin drop, eat too much and too fast before we notice what we are tasting, or suck air with flaring nostrils to smell the delicate aroma of a flower.

How could it be any other way? Nowadays most of us live in what are commonly called "stressful" environments—loud, fast, tight, pressured. Often it seems that the only way to survive and keep up is to also be loud, fast, and pressured. This cyclic pattern of stress creating stress is what causes dis-stress in our bodies and minds.

It seems strange to think that when the Buddha taught the First Noble Truth—that suffering exists—he could have understood so long ago the gapless intensity of our current times, but it's all relative. Gautama Shakyamuni lived in India during a time of rapid city growth and the culture was shifting toward urban development. Time and space were shrinking then just as now. Whenever your situation becomes faster, tighter, and more condensed, the quality of claustrophia creates an environment of discomfort, a state of *dis*ease and distress.

Growing up in the 1960s I remember my parents talking over the dinner table about so-and-so having this illness, and that person having another illness, and all of these problems being a result of "stress." My parents said, "Oh, the doctors these days say everything comes from stress!" Well, now we know that chronic stress does create profound physical disturbances, such as increases in heart rate, blood pressure, and muscle tension. In many cases, stress *is* what causes illness, and it's becoming more common every day.

Being a yoga teacher I am fascinated by people's bodies—their posture and physical anatomy; the way they move through space; and the harmony or disharmony of their energy. I'm not interested in discovering what fashionistas would consider the size, shape, and proportions of a "perfect body"—it's how they are all working together that intrigues me. Is there a graceful balance of body, mind, and breath? Is the rhythm of the body staccato or legato; allegro, andante, or moderato? Is there support for the breath or do the ribs look like they were stuck onto the waist and hips by a kindergartner with a bottle of Elmer's Glue?

Being a yoga teacher in New York is especially fun because I see a wide variety of bodies negotiating their way through the busy, noisy streets. We might have different fitness levels, backgrounds, religions, and politics, but one thing New Yorkers have in common is a body-clenching experience every time a city bus backfires.

Decibels make a difference. I asked my composer husband to demonstrate a decibel for me and he said, "A decibel is a measurement equal to a hair." He went on to explain that a decibel can be heard by the sensitive ear of a music professional but for others, although it cannot be heard, it is still felt. Did you know that when you hold two musical tuning forks and hit one, as it begins to tone, the other fork will ring in response without even being touched? This is the same thing that happens to our bones when we are near a jackhammer. Even if you don't live in a big city, you may still have the same bone-knocking response to the sound of the coffee bean grinder in your kitchen.

Many of us exist in this semipermanent body fist. Inside, our nervous system also jumps up a notch until eventually we are living in a fairly continuous state of pumped-up adrenaline. This condition is called fight-or-flight, and it is very helpful if you are walking in the woods and encounter a bear. When we are under attack, our mind tells our body to relate to an emergency and our body responds by kicking in the adrenal glands, which tell our heart to pump faster, raising blood pressure, increasing muscle tension, and producing sweat. Our metabolism shifts in order to store more energy, causing less immediate issues such as digestion, growth, and reproduction to close up shop temporarily. This helps us have the energy and mental alertness necessary to deal with threatening situations.

The natural pattern that follows an emergency situation is exhaustion because extra energy has been used. Remaining in a fight-or-flight condition for an extended period of time leads to *dis*ease, a.k.a. stress or dis-stress. Over time you start to fatigue more easily, increase your risk of diabetes, raise your blood pressure, and become at risk for peptic ulcers and reproductive disorders. Remember how the fight-or-flight condition tells your systems of digestion, reproduction, growth, and repair to slow down? If you end up on this plateau, it is obviously going to create health problems.

Even if we tell ourselves to relax, we are so wound up that we can't. The warm refuge of the bed might look inviting but may not support your kidneys, lower back, heart, lungs, or brain in a way that is conducive to rejuvenation. The answering machine, the digital alarm clock light, the neighbor's dog, the neighbors—there are many light and sound intrusions on what used to be a completely quiet blackout time. So we have insomnia, we toss and turn, we get too hot or too cold, the mattress cover bunches up under our kidneys, and nightmares torture us.

Unfortunately we are using up our store of extra fight-or-flight energy day and night and for no reason except that our bodies are trying to protect us from the onslaught of noise, job overload, personal transitions, and traffic jams of all sorts. That's why most of us collapse in a heap on the couch the first chance we get. We understand active and we understand passive. It is crucial that we learn to live in the middle of these two dysfunctional extremes.

LEARNING TO RECEIVE

The brilliance of yoga relaxation technique is that it combines what we already know—the active quality of tadasana, mountain pose, and the passive quality of savasana, corpse pose, which leads to the middle path that combines the best of the two—the ability to be receptive.

The foundation of all standing asanas is tadasana, or mountain pose. The mindful actions of extending out through the leg and arm bones as you pull the muscles up toward your center; engaging the pelvic floor in conversation between pubic bone and tailbone; and continuously exploring the internal and external rotation of the limbs in order to support the pelvis, spine, and shoulder girdle can be applied to every asana. This requires a vibrancy and attentiveness that is invigorating and informative. Standing in tadasana is like coming to attention, not in a military way, but by aligning your mind with your body.

Savasana means corpse pose and is practice for the moment when we will actually die and leave our physical body but maintain awareness of our mind stream. This profound level of release—even letting go of our body identity—is what is cultivated through the practice of savasana. Savasana is the base for all supine poses in yoga, including all restorative yoga postures.

Combining the "coming to attention" quality of tadasana with the complete physical "letting go" of savasana leads us to this middle path quality of "coming to our senses" which is found in being receptive. In yoga, the opposite of active is not passive, but receptive. The ability to stay aware of the richness of each moment, but content to experience it without needing to change, control, or manage it.

On a deep level, restorative yoga balances our masculine and feminine aspects of outgo and input, space and form, light and dark, dominant and submissive, active and passive. The experience of relaxed wakefulness in both body and mind can only be found by being receptive. If you push too hard, you will miss it. If you fall asleep you will miss it, too.

Restorative yoga is not a fancy way of taking a nap nor is it stretching, which can easily become another way to generate craving, which is definitely not relaxing. Instead of *doing* yoga, this form of yoga *does* us. Restorative asana practice provides a framework for openings of body, breath, and mind to occur naturally over time, without tightening, stretching, or collapsing. Through precise placement of props such as blankets and cushions, one establishes an environment that promotes physical and mental relaxation. Placing your body in these positions is like creating a map for the internal rivers of blood, breath, water, and energy to follow. This will nourish your abdominal organs, rest your muscles, and balance your hormones, as well as soothe the nervous system, which, in turn, calms the mind.

As your body is reprogrammed to reduce brain arousal, fluid retention, adrenal burnout, and toxic buildup, your mind is invited to watch the process. Restorative yoga is not a magic bed that lets you sleep and guarantees perfect health when you wake up. It is a practice that creates a strong possibility for a certain response, but no promise when that will happen or how it will show up. That's why you have to stay awake. What is happening is subtle and profound, but you will miss it if you fall asleep or space out.

Sometimes people try to stop their minds altogether and freeze up as a result, just like I did when my date told me to relax. Trying to suppress the contents of one's mind and create a certain state of relaxation is still an activity. Restorative yoga suggests that we can even relax our idea of what we want to get from this exercise and simply pay attention to what it feels like to be oneself in this physical configuration. Letting go of what we want from this practice, or from anything else we do, is a huge step toward feeling relaxed, restored, rejuvenated. Rather than accomplishing only one goal, this approach provides endless possibility for opening to occur in every level of our being.

Observe the movements of your mind with a light touch and friendly awareness. Don't try to stop thoughts and don't get caught up in them. You may find that the physical positions of the restorative asanas themselves naturally slow down your thoughts, but if not, that's fine. Notice your experience without any judgment.

At first it might seem like these restorative poses are not as valuable as more active asana practice, and it is difficult to take the time to do them. It took a while for restorative yoga to catch on at OM. In truth, it is an advanced practice. The subtlety of the experience, the necessary mindfulness, the patience to wait for your body, mind, and breath to unfold on their own schedule, is not always available to a beginning yogi. Usually an advanced practitioner might even have to hit bottom energetically before understanding the value of this sophisticated practice. Restorative yoga was welcomed on September 25, 2001, when I taught a sold-out benefit class to raise money for the firefighters of New York City.

In the face of the world's instability, it is not surprising that we have lost confidence in the earth to hold us up. In restorative yoga we attempt to regain that confidence by bringing the earth up to meet us with small piles of pillows and blankets. In each pose, check to make sure that every part of your body feels supported by having a cushion or blanket under the curves of your body. That is crucial to restorative work. Keeping your joints in flexion gives us the feeling of being held, which is a big part of what allows us to let go on a deep, subconscious level.

Well-known restorative yoga teacher Jane Fryer calls her workshops "Body Holiday." Try to give your body a mini holiday as often as you can. The recommendation is:

- Once a day include twenty minutes of restorative yoga in your practice.

- Once a week make your full yoga practice be completely restorative—Sunday is nice for that.

- Once a year make your yoga practice be restorative every day for a week—this is nice in the winter when the earth goes quiet, too.

If just thinking about doing this makes you stress out, then don't think about it. Just do it when you can and let the feelings that arise from the practice be your guide. Over time you will find that you look forward to those twenty minutes, which, rather than being another thing to fit into your busy schedule, somehow create even more time and space in your day. As you create the conditions for your body to open, the practice will create the conditions for your life to open.

CONSCIOUS RESTING

Savasana, conscious resting, is an exercise unique to yoga, and one of the secrets of why this form of physical training works. In addition to physical benefits such as lowering blood pressure, enhancing the immune system, calming the nervous system, and releasing muscular effort, the lesson of learning how to relax with awareness, without falling asleep or going unconscious, may be the most profound.

As part of the teacher training program at OM Yoga Center, each student is required to observe several yoga classes, which always include savasana at the end. The teacher trainees never fail to be moved at the sight of a room full of people, especially New Yorkers, trusting enough to lie on their backs with their eyes closed, unmoving, for at least ten minutes. The ability to remain quiet, let go into the earth, and be that exposed, takes bravery, confidence, and letting go—the bravery to look inside yourself; the confidence that what you will learn about yourself is basically good; the ability to let go of whatever comes up and still stay open, quiet, and grounded. This is called savasana, corpse pose, and it is when we learn not to do, but to be.

Many people find it difficult to relax, slow down, stop doing. For them it is more challenging to "let go" than just "go." Even if you have not done a yoga class you can always do corpse pose in lieu of a nap when you need to rejuvenate in a spacious and alert way. You may find it to be more effective for resting body and mind than napping because it has a structure that aids physical and mental release.

Here are the basic instructions for corpse pose.

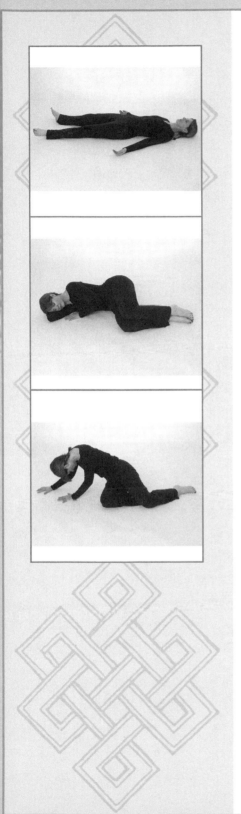

SAVASANA (CORPSE POSE)

Lie down with your back on the floor. If the floor is not warm, put a blanket underneath you.

Let your legs lie naturally, with your feet about hip distance apart. If your legs are too close together, your abdominal muscles will not release. If they are too wide apart, your outer hips won't release.

Place your arms about eight to ten inches from the sides of your body. If your arms are too close to your body, your shoulders will be tense. If your arms are too far out, you will have a subconscious level of vulnerability that will not allow you to relax. Turn your palms to face upward, creating external rotation in the arms to support the heart and lungs.

If your lower back feels uncomfortable, place a rolled-up blanket or towel under your knees. If your chin is closer to the ceiling than your forehead, place a small pillow or blanket under the base of your skull, to soften and lengthen the back of your neck.

Cover yourself with a blanket if you think you might get cold.

Close your eyes. Place an eye pillow over your eyes, if you like.

Let your breathing be completely natural. Watch your thoughts coming and going like clouds floating through the sky. Recognize the sky as your mind.

Stay like this for five to ten minutes.

To come out of corpse pose, begin to deepen your breathing. Can you enjoy the feeling of the breath running through your body? Make small movements with your toes and fingers. Softly bend your knees and roll over onto your

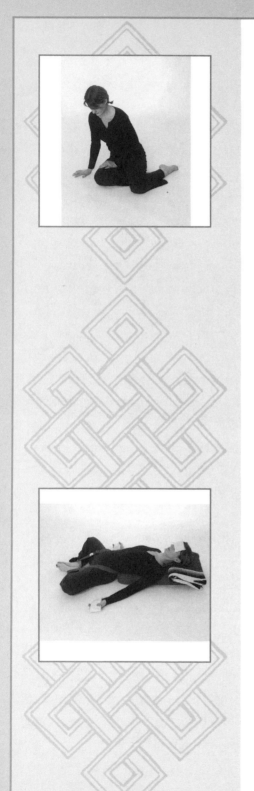

right side. (The left side of the body is the feminine aspect and when you roll to the right, you allow the channel of receptivity, quiet, cooling to open further.) Use your right arm as a pillow and rest here for a minute or so. When you are ready, use your hands to slowly walk yourself back up to sitting. Let your head dangle and be the last thing to come up to maintain the quality of relaxation as you come back to vertical.

No matter how long or short, make sure you complete every asana practice with savasana. Just as we learn to balance forward bends with backward bends, we learn to balance effort with noneffort, doing and not-doing.

Yoga Body

RESTORATIVE YOGA SEQUENCE

1. Supported Bound Angle Pose
This pose is a wonderful hip and chest opener. Take your time to get set up just right so you can really relax in this powerful pose. This is good for anybody, anytime, but particularly welcome during menstruation and menopause. In addition to eye pillows on your eyes, anytime you are in a reclining restorative pose you can put eye pillows in your palms, which feels comforting and helps one drop even more into the lap of the earth.

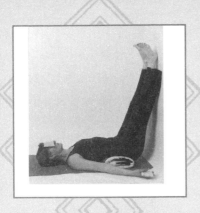

2. Legs up the Wall Pose

Neatly fold one or two blankets. Place your lower back on the blankets with your sitting bones between the blanket and the wall. You can experiment with how close to the wall you want your bottom to be. For people with tighter hamstrings and low backs, you will be happier a little farther away from the wall. Place another small rolled-up blanket under your neck and slightly under your shoulders. A pillow under your head can be used to elevate your forehead higher than your chin without constricting your throat.

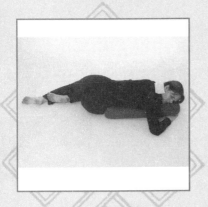

3. Twist

Place the blankets or bolster at your right hip. Press down on the bolster as you lengthen your ribs up off your pelvis, getting long in the waist. As you exhale, twist to the right and lie down on the bolster. You can turn your head either way. To come out of the pose, use your hands to walk yourself up to sitting. Shift your knees over to the left and you are ready to twist to the other side.

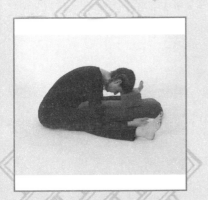

4. Supported Forward Bend

You may need to use several blankets and bolsters to get the support you need for this pose. You can also try it on a stool, chair seat, or the back of a chair. It's also nice to pile up blankets under your chest, so when you bend forward you are fully supported and can relax here. If you have a tight lower back or hamstrings, place a small blanket or cushion under your sitting bones, just as you would in any seated forward bend. Restorative yoga is not about stretching but about letting go and opening. If that is not your experience, reorganize your setup so that it supports you.

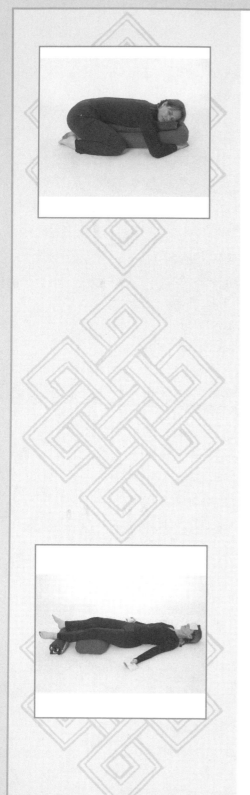

5. Supported Child's Pose

Place two to four neatly folded blankets lengthwise and fold your body over them. If you have a carpet, you don't need a blanket under your shins. Your torso should be completely supported by the blankets and your thighs. If it's not, then you need more blankets. Wrap your arms around the blankets just as you would wrap them around your bed pillows. Turn your head to one side, and after a while turn it to the other side. It's also nice to place a little eye pillow on your lower back to help lengthen that area.

6. Supported Corpse Pose

This pose will be familiar to you as the same one you do when you are floating on a swimming pool raft or resting on a chaise lounge. That cellular memory alone may help you begin to relax. This pose is particularly good for enhancing breathing and for opening the heart center. Place the lengthwise folded blankets just below your waist and lie back on them. Once again, your forehead should be slightly higher than your chin, with a soft, open throat and free breathing.

7. Corpse Pose

You can do simple corpse pose or you can add blankets under the chest, head, and knees. (Pictured on page 235.)

TWELVE

CREATING THE MANDALA

How to Frame Your Practice

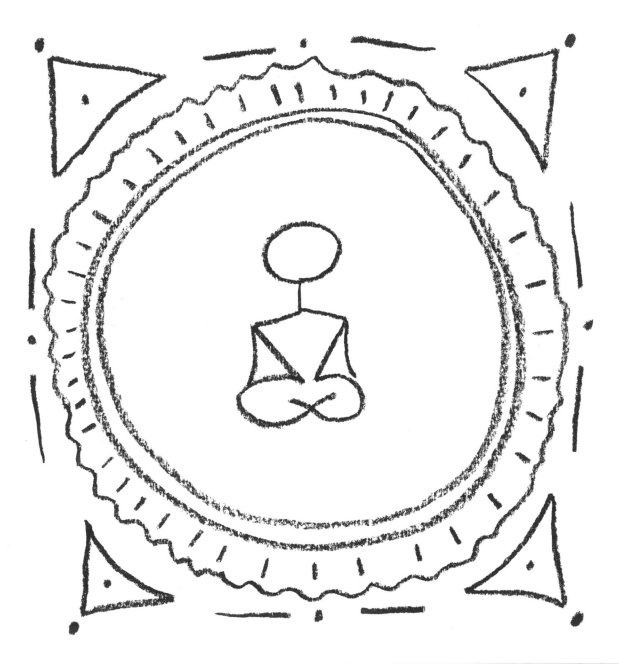

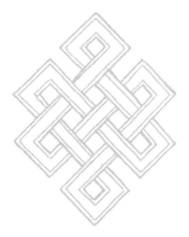

PRECISION, BOUNDARIES, NO BIG DEAL

Before you begin your practice it is important to establish a supportive environment. This is called creating the mandala, or sacred space and time to practice yoga and meditation. Traditionally it refers to an arrangement of energy with a center and boundaries.

First, get organized. Gather your practice materials in one place so you don't have to leave the room, which will disrupt your flow and tempt you to do other things. Bring your yoga mat, a blanket or two, eye pillow, meditation cushion, yoga belt or block, and any other practical items into your practice area. Place your mat and props in a neat arrangement. By doing this you may begin to understand how form creates space. Just as you work with precise alignment, be precise in how you set up an environment to enable a spacious experience. You may wish to include natural elements such as flowers, incense, or fire in the form of candles, to shift the energy of the room. Other than that, it doesn't have to be a big deal.

One of the main elements of a mandala is the protector principle, which maintains the sacredness of the space and time for you while you are there. In some Japanese temples the protectors are huge scary-looking statues of demon-like gods with fangs and claws standing at the entrance. In our case, the protectors can be very basic actions to establish boundaries. These actions could include sweeping the floor, turning off your cell phone, asking your family not to bother you, making a commitment to staying with your practice for a specific length of time.

Sometimes we feel we can't even get started because we don't have the right outfit or a big enough space or the right floor or enough time. Don't let these details become obstacles. The situation will never be perfect, and yet, it is always just right. The space becomes sacred when you enter it with the pure intention to connect to yourself. Can you be curious to what might happen? Can you be honest? Try to recognize the benefits you are cultivating and dedicate your efforts for the benefit of all beings.

CHANTING OM

OM is a mantra, or vibration, that is traditionally chanted at the beginning and end of yoga sessions. It is a primordial sound that is said to be the sound of the universe. What does that mean?

Somehow the ancient yogis knew what our scientists today are telling us—that the entire universe is moving. Nothing is ever solid or still. Everything that exists pulsates, creating a rhythmic vibration that the ancient yogis acknowledged with the sound of OM. We may not always be aware of this sound in our daily lives but we can hear it in the rustling of the autumn leaves, the waves on the shore, the flutter of a bird's wings, the inside of a seashell.

Chanting OM allows us to listen to the rhythm of our own breath and recognize our experience as a reflection of how the whole universe moves—the setting sun, the rising moon, the ebb and flow of the tides, and the beating of our hearts. We are reminded of the impermanence of everything, and the preciousness of each moment of our life. As we chant OM, it takes us for a ride on this universal movement, through our breath, our awareness, and our physical energy, and we begin to sense a bigger connection that is both uplifting and soothing. This is the true meaning of yoga.

OM is made up of four parts: A, U, M, and the silence at the end. As you chant these sounds, you will notice how the A evolves into the U to make the sound of O. Linger on the M as you finish your exhale. Let your mind ride out on your breath and mix with the silent space, the gap, at the end of OM.

Chant OM three times at the beginning and end of your practice. If you feel too shy to chant it out loud, you can do it in your mind.

DEDICATING THE BENEFITS

When we breathe consciously, we are aware of both the inhalation and the exhalation. One of my pranayama teachers said that we are born knowing how to inhale, but we have to learn to exhale, to let go, to be generous. Just as that cycle is only complete through both the receiving and the giving actions of the breath, our practice is really only complete when we dedicate our practice. This means that we acknowledge the positivity of our good-hearted efforts, and instead of trying to hold on to that, allowing it to ferment, we continue the circulation of that energy by sending it back out to all beings.

This practice is powerful because it is a commitment to sharing your benefits with ALL BEINGS EVERYWHERE, not just the people you know and love. This dedication prayer is called the Four Immeasurables. It is a big open-heart practice where you send your merit out to an immeasurable number of beings—including humans, animals, fish, birds, even cockroaches—all the beings that you love, those you don't like, and the many, many beings you will never even meet.

I learned this prayer from my teacher, Gehlek Rimpoche, and found it to be transformative in my life. It is simple but strong. Eventually I began to say it out loud at the end of my yoga classes with no intention other than to dedicate the merit at that time. One day, the whole class joined me. It was an amazing, spontaneous moment. This genuine heart offering from all the students has continued and now we say this dedication at the end of every class at OM Yoga Center.

Anyone can make this intention. You do not have to be a Buddhist to wish others happiness. If you like, at the end of your practice, take a moment to say the following prayer and dedicate whatever positive merit may have arisen from your endeavors today to the benefit of all beings. Like inhaling and exhaling, we assimilate the effects of our meditation and yoga practice—open body, open mind, open heart—and radiate them out to others, connecting once again to the pulsation of everything and everyone everywhere.

May all beings have happiness and the causes of happiness.
May all beings be free from suffering and the causes of suffering.
May all beings never be parted from freedom's true joy.
May all beings dwell in equanimity, free from attachment and aversion.

CONCLUSION

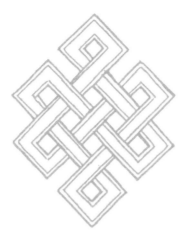

PROCESS

Several years ago I slipped in late to a dharma talk, and found a seat in the back row next to an old friend I hadn't seen for years. It took a moment for her to recognize me and then she said, "Oh! You look different. You're more processed." My first reaction was "Processed? Blah. Ick." But I couldn't stop thinking about that comment and I've thought about it ever since then. What did she see? Am I processed and boring like Velveeta cheese? Is that bad? Maybe that's equanimity. Have I become mellow or refined? Has my enthusiasm for the dharma waned? Has an ability to be patient kicked in, even a little bit?

I don't know what she saw but I do know what I feel, which is profoundly grateful for being introduced to the practices of yoga and meditation. I don't always feel relaxed or patient or kind or confident or generous or spacious. But sometimes I do, and I know those moments of clarity will come again if I stay connected to my practices.

At this point I've lost my craving to accomplish the fanciest, biggest, most upside-down poses every day, and my desire to be a perfect posture supergirl meditator has passed. I've learned not to look for a specific experience or answer that can be held or even relied on. What I do work on is my commitment to practice because I know for sure that the process is what holds the key to all the benefits of yoga and meditation practice.

When you make a commitment like this, your daily practice of meditation and yoga is called a sadhana. Sadhana comes from the word *saddha*, which means faith. Rather than any guarantees to hang our faith on, we are invited to have faith in the process. We learn to trust that although the results of our commitment are sometimes invisible or ineffable, they are there and they are beneficial.

One of my students had a heart attack in his early forties. After a year of slowly recuperating and rebuilding his strength through cardiovascular activity, he began taking the Brand-New Beginner yoga series at my studio, OM Yoga Center. On September 11, 2001, he was on his morning jog in New York's Riverside Park when he heard a loud explosive sound and thought he was having another heart attack. He immediately remembered the calming breath technique he had learned in yoga class and was able to regain some composure. Looking down the river, he saw smoke and realized that the sound he had heard was the collapse of the first World Trade Center tower. He felt that yoga saved his life that day. He wasn't strong or flexible yet, but the benefit of his one yoga class was an ability to control his breath—and therefore his mind and nervous system—which softened the fear and panic that might have hurt his heart again.

Some of the benefits of practice are more immediate and tangible than others. I think of a yoga body as strong, well-functioning, clean inside and out. Buddha mind means an alert, spacious, kind mind . . . and heart. Through our practice this is what we are cultivating but I can't even guarantee that to you.

Although I know I have a strong and fluid body, sometimes I feel weak, tired, dry, tight, and bored. I have been known to be cranky and selfish. At those times I certainly do not feel like meditating because who wants to look at their mind when it feels like that? And how can I be enthusiastic about yoga when I feel bloated? I do it anyway. Feeling enthusiastic is not a requirement. Doing it is a requirement.

That's where the commitment to the process comes in. Feeling gung-ho or not becomes irrelevant. That's just how it is today. Or right in this moment. It will change in the next five minutes. In fact, I am quite sure that after five breaths on the cushion and three sun salutations I will feel different. That unfolding, and the awareness of it, is what holds my interest and keeps me coming back to practice rather than any specific idea of what might be gained. I've learned that some days I might float, or swim, or even sink a little bit, but because of my practices I have the courage and confidence to more fully fall into the river of life without drowning or holding my breath.

In this way, learning to take interest in the process of my own life has led to deeper curiosity and caring about others. Science tells us that when a butterfly flaps its wings today, it creates a rainstorm on the other side of the world tomorrow. Medicine tells us that when we get even a tiny scrape on our elbow, our entire body goes to work to heal it. All energy is interrelated and everything works together. We might not have the ability to control the outcome of things but we can be mindful of how our own thoughts, words, and actions affect others. The understanding that we are practicing not just for our own well-being but for that of the whole world is the most profound benefit of practice.

Yoga philosophy says that our body is a map of the entire universe. Pema Chödron says that when we practice meditation we are studying humanity in the form of ourselves. When we understand that our body is part of the whole world's body and our mind is part of the whole world's mind, we understand the true meaning of Yoga Body, Buddha Mind—strong, vast, and all-inclusive.

This sounds very grand but we don't have to be heroic. We can be ordinary mothers and fathers, teachers, accountants, plumbers, lawyers, grocers, decorators, musicians, ministers, and potters—all of us learning to take interest in our own unfolding. As we become more able to feel what comes up in our heart we can let that be the key to harmonizing our mind/intentions with our body/actions. It doesn't require grand gestures. Just simply attending to each moment.

Good luck.

CLASS PROGRAMS

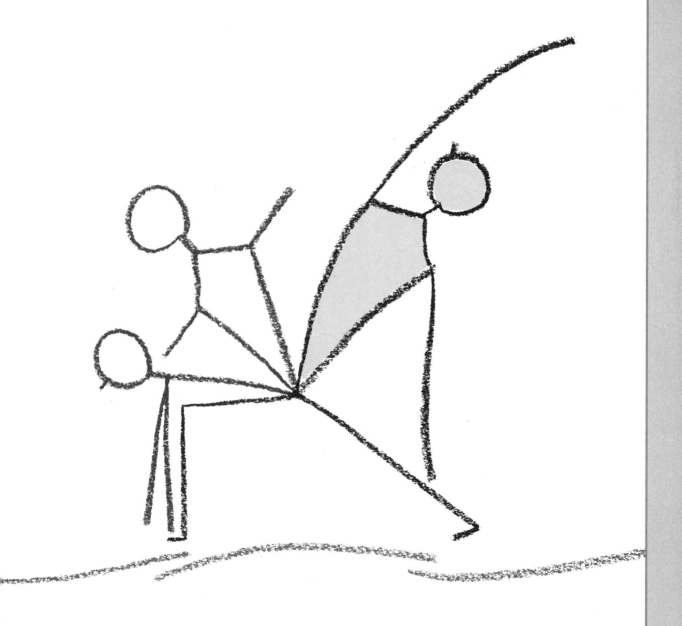

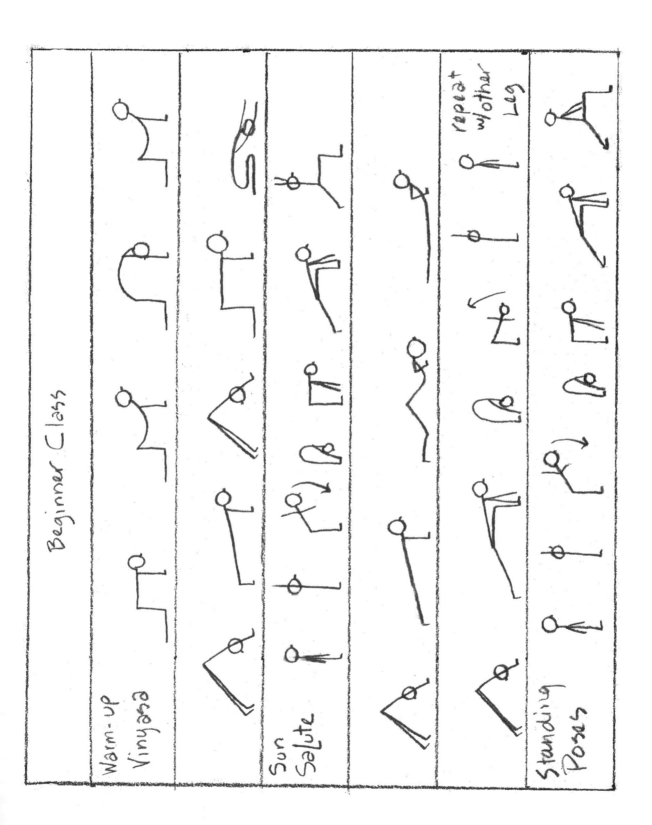

Beginner Class

Warm-up
Vinyasa

Sun
Salute

repeat
w/other
Leg

Standing
Poses

Beginner Class continued

repeat standing poses on other side to here, then continue

do this much on the other side, then

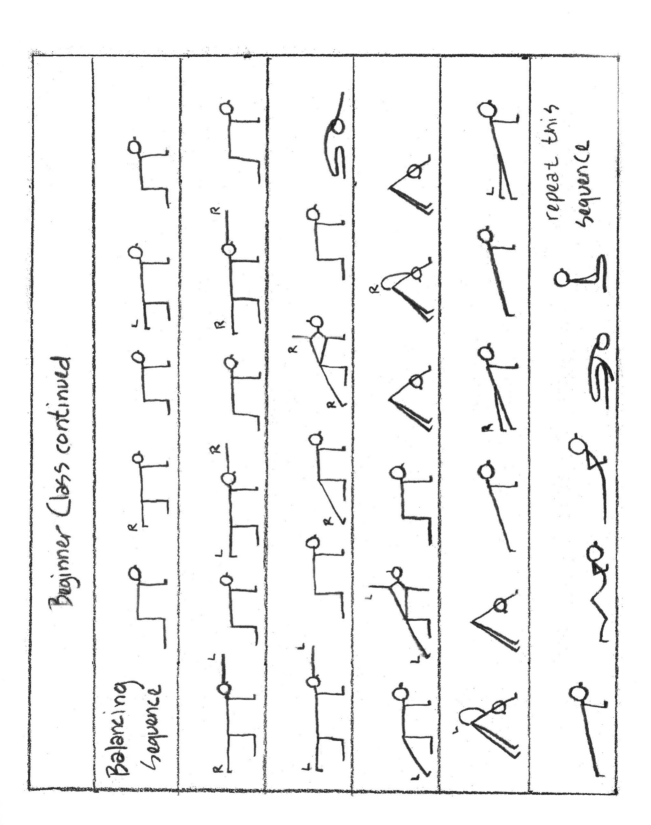

Beginner Class continued

Balancing Sequence

repeat this sequence

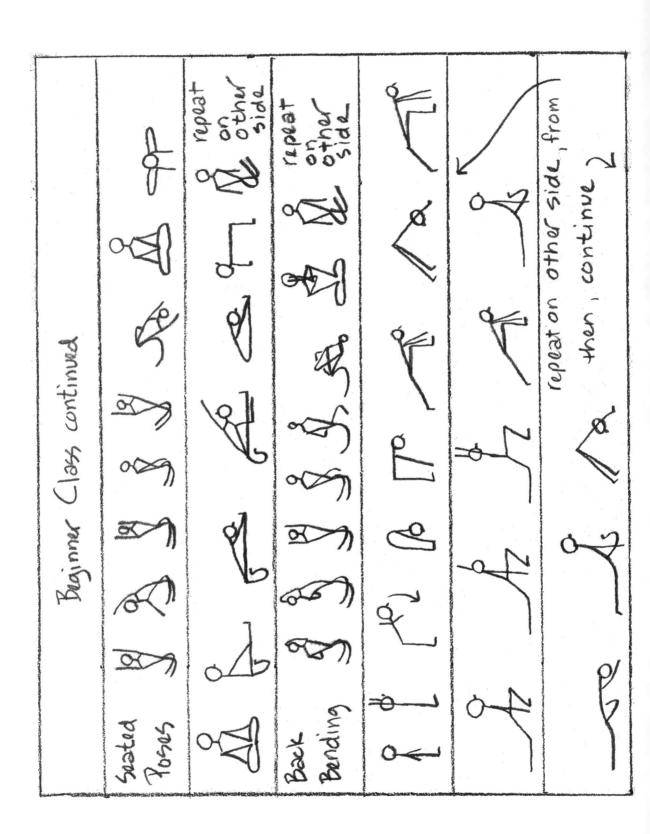

Beginner Class continued

Seated Poses

repeat on other side

Back Bending

repeat on other side

repeat on other side, from then, continue

Beginner Class continued.

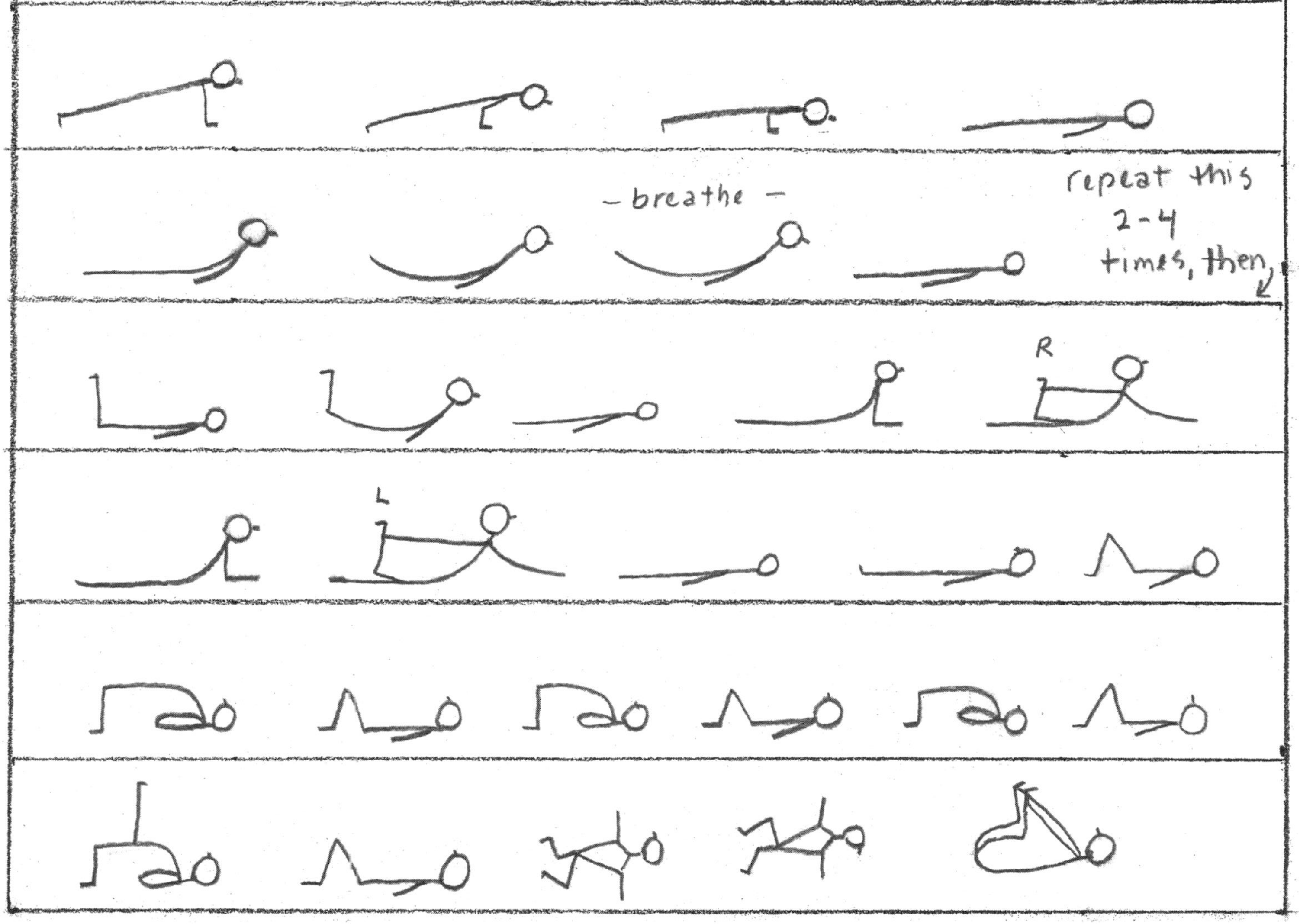

repeat this
2-4
times, then,

— breathe —

R

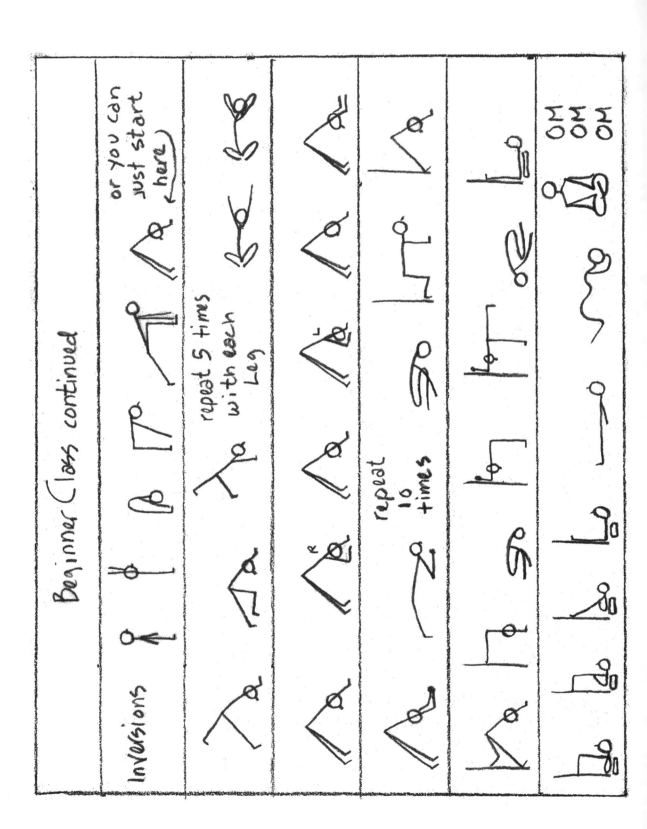

Beginner Class continued

Inversions

or you can just start here

repeat 5 times with each Leg

repeat 10 times

OM
OM
OM

Intermediate Class

Calming Breath	Inhale for 5 counts — OM Exhale for 5 counts — OM repeat for 3-5 minutes — OM

Warm-up vinyasa

Sun Salute

or

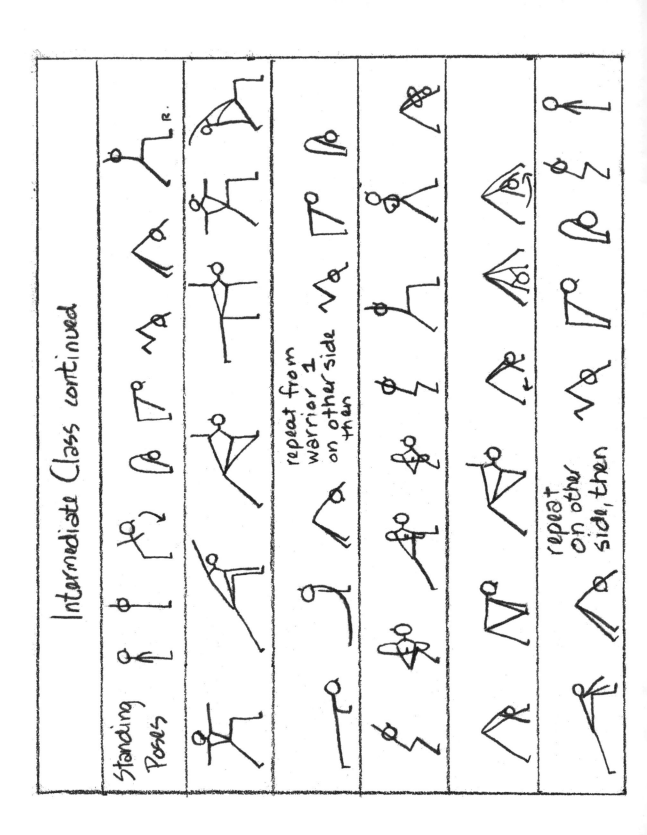

Intermediate Class continued

Standing Poses

repeat from
warrior 1
on other side
then

repeat
on other
side, then

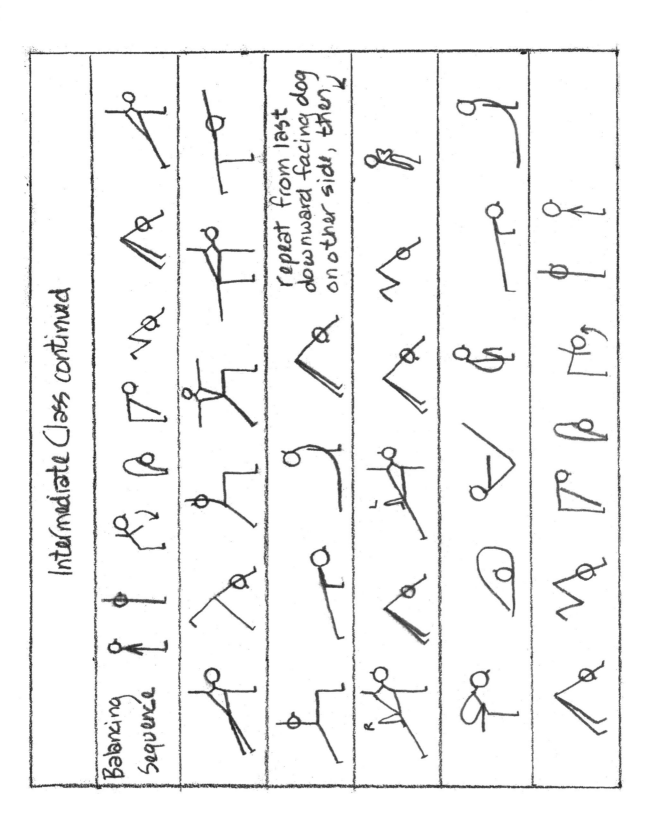

Intermediate Class continued

Balancing Sequence

repeat from last downward facing dog on other side, then

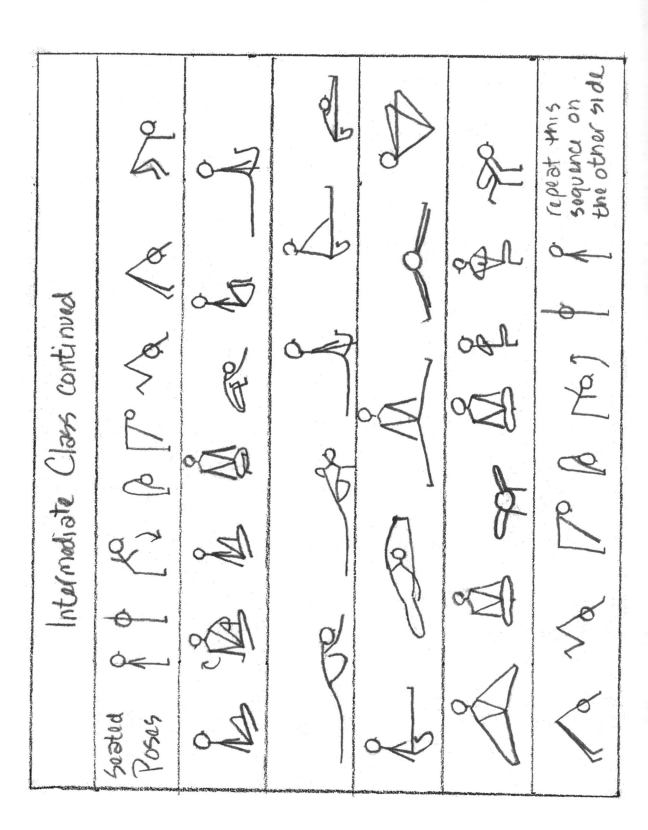

Intermediate Class continued

Seated Poses

repeat this sequence on the other side

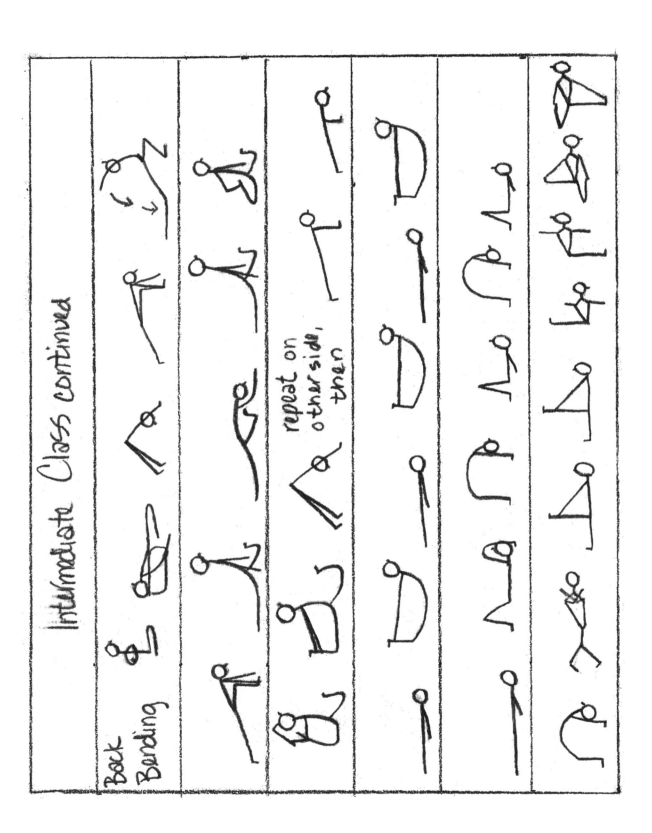

Intermediate Class continued

Back Bending

repeat on other side, then

Intermediate Class continued

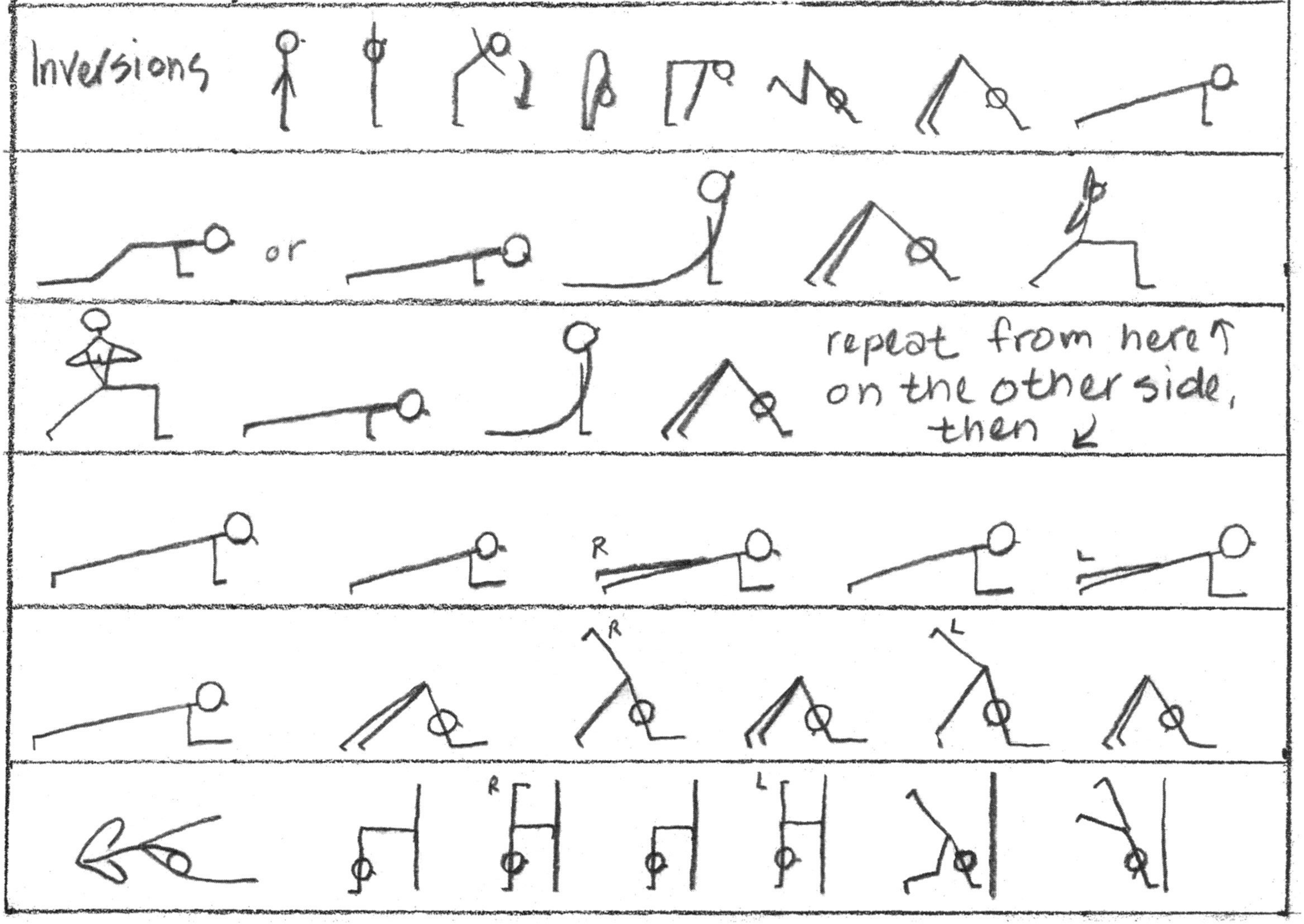
Inversions
or
repeat from here ↑
on the other side,
then ↙
R
L
R
L
R
L

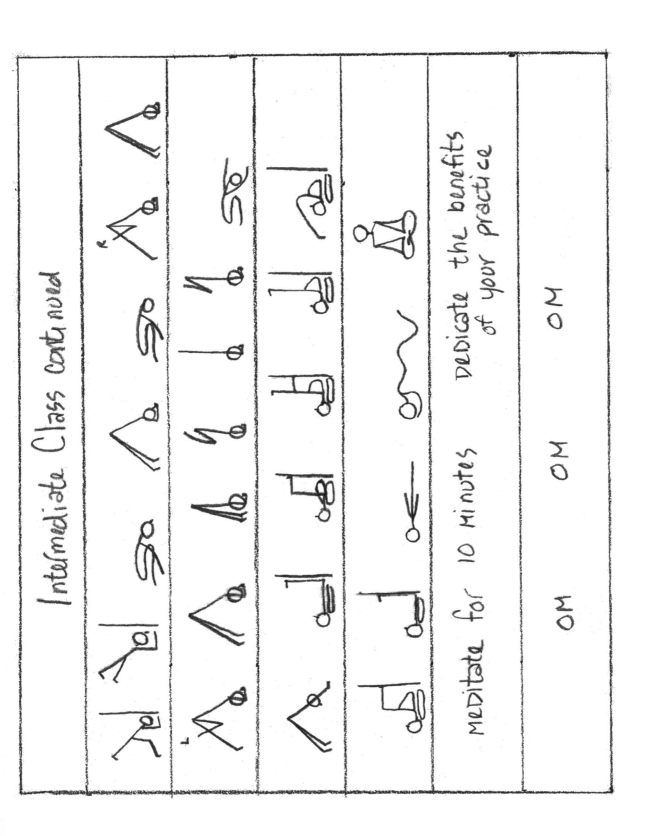

Intermediate Class continued

Meditate for 10 minutes   Dedicate the benefits of your practice

OM   OM   OM

Advanced Class

Alternate Nostril Breathing	Calming or Breath	Sitting Meditation
		OM OM OM

Warm-up Vinyasa (variation)

Sun Salute

Standing Poses

Advanced Class continued

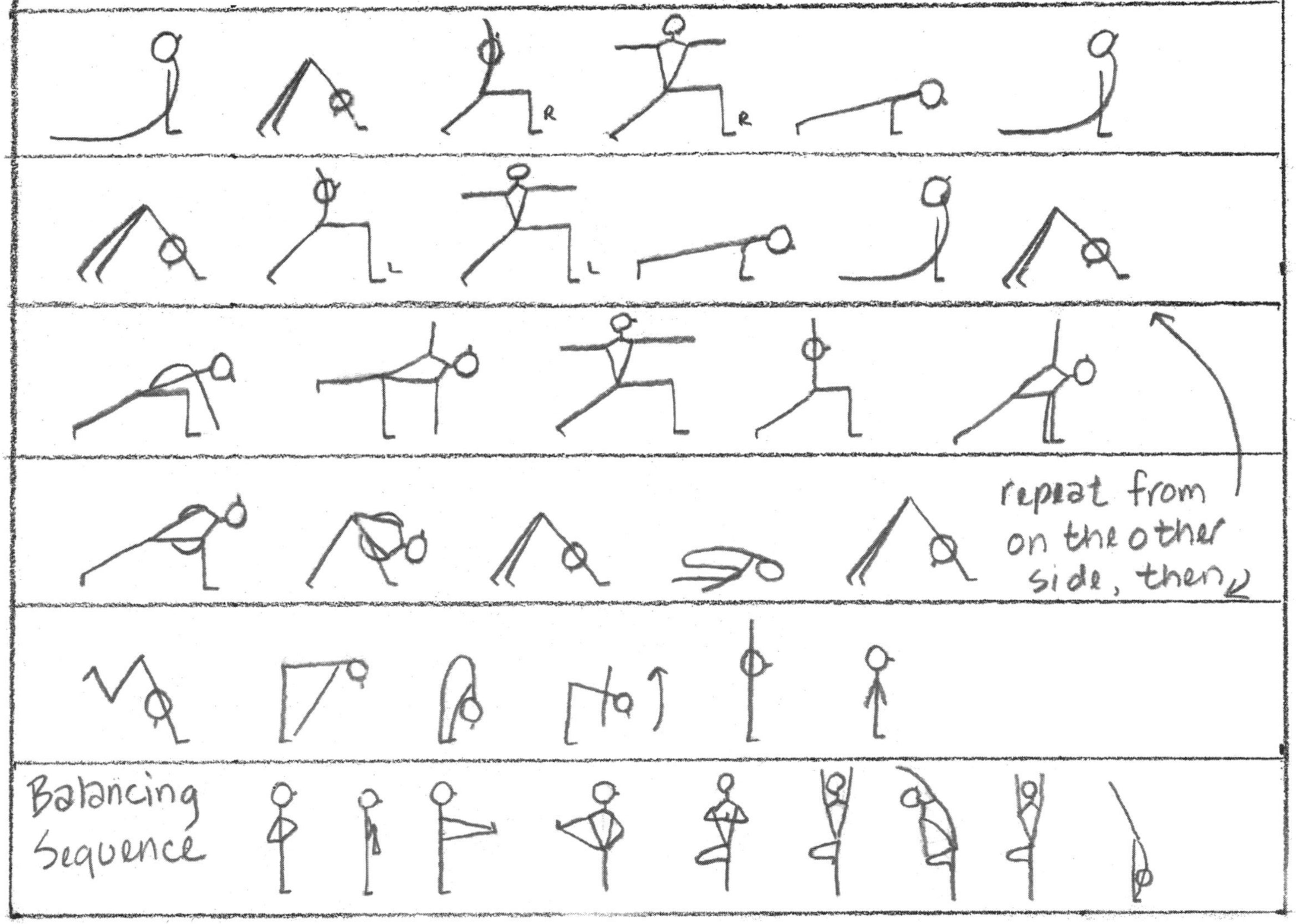

repeat from
on the other
side, then

Balancing
Sequence

Advanced Class continued

Advanced Class continued

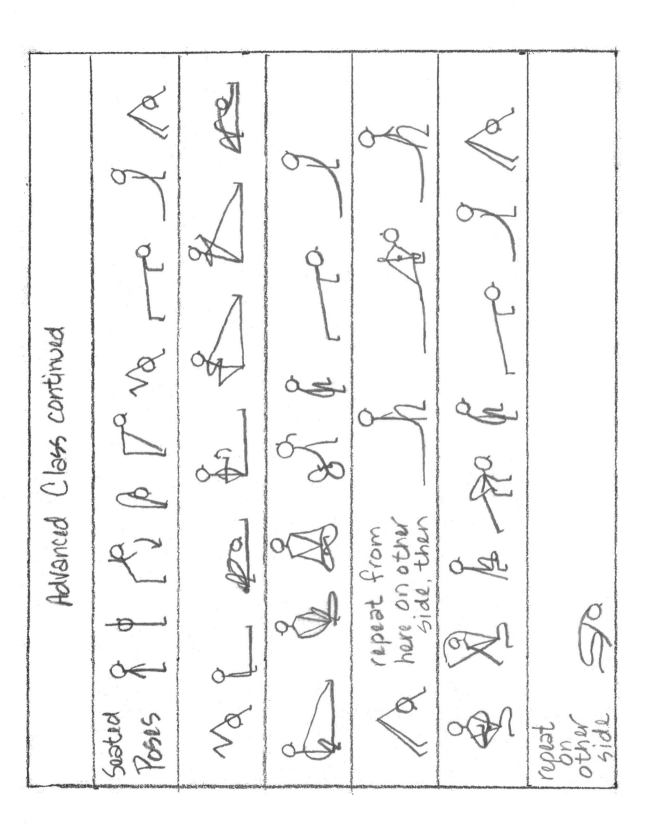

Seated Poses

repeat from here on other side, then

repeat on other side

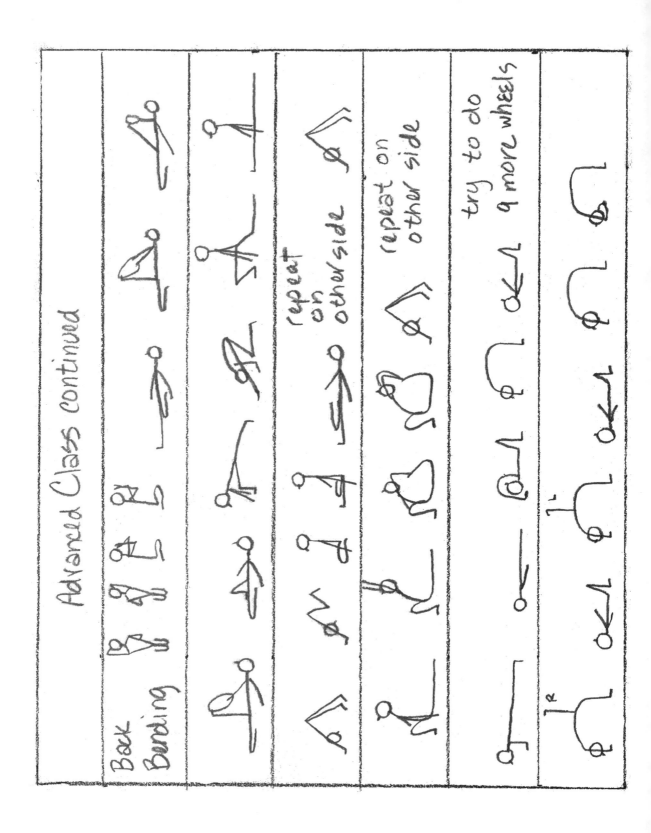

Advanced Class continued

Back Bending

repeat on otherside

repeat on other side

try to do 9 more wheels

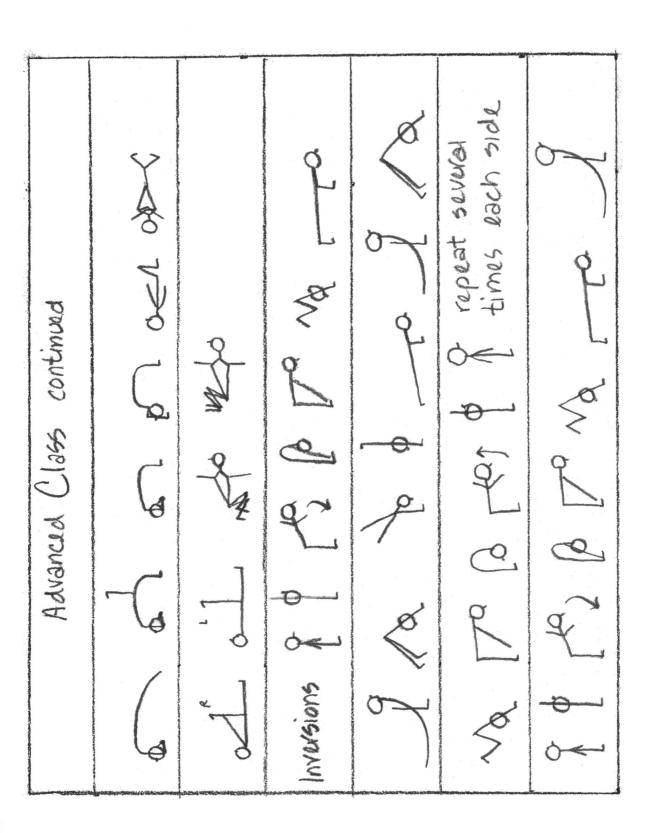

Advanced Class continued

Inversions

repeat several
times each side

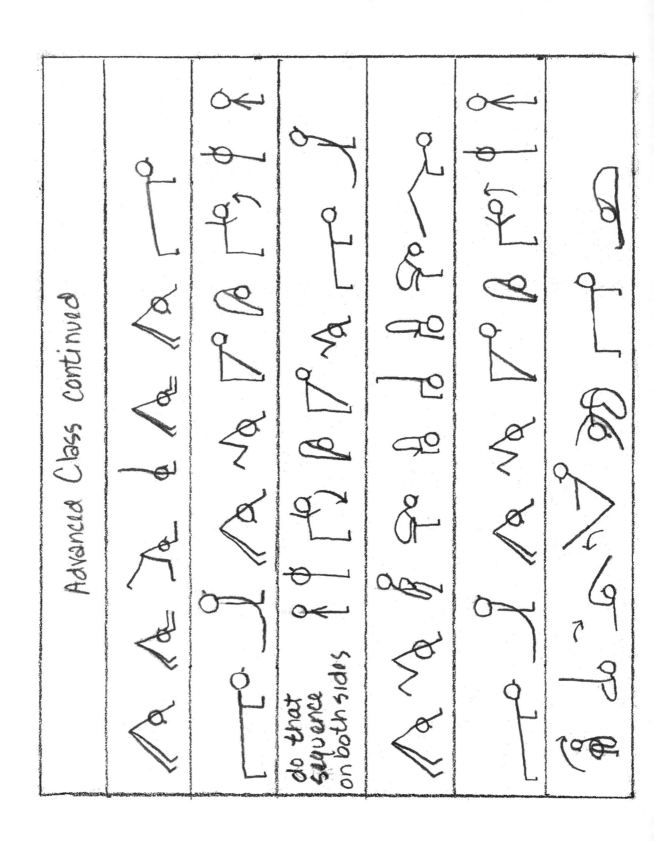

Advanced Class Continued

do that
sequence
on both sides

Advanced Class continued

repeat a few times

or try:

Sitting Meditation

Dedicate your Practice

OM   OM   OM

OM